From Mr. Suri
Blackpool victoria Hospital
Sep 2022.

SNIPPETS IN
SURGERY
VOL 1

ILLUSTRATED ESSENTIALS
OF GENERAL SURGERY

SRINIVASAN RAVI

BALBOA.PRESS
A DIVISION OF HAY HOUSE

Balboa Press books may be ordered through booksellers or by contacting:

Balboa Press
A Division of Hay House
1663 Liberty Drive
Bloomington, IN 47403
www.balboapress.co.uk
UK TFN: 0800 0148647 (Toll Free inside the UK)
UK Local: (02) 0369 56325 (+44 20 3695 6325 from outside the UK)

Because of the dynamic nature of the Internet, any web addresses or links contained in this book may have changed since publication and may no longer be valid. The views expressed in this work are solely those of the author and do not necessarily reflect the views of the publisher, and the publisher hereby disclaims any responsibility for them.

The author of this book does not dispense medical advice or prescribe the use of any technique as a form of treatment for physical, emotional, or medical problems without the advice of a physician, either directly or indirectly. The intent of the author is only to offer information of a general nature to help you in your quest for emotional and spiritual well-being. This is a surgical book and I am not catering to any one's spirituality. In the event you use any of the information in this book for yourself, which is your constitutional right, the author and the publisher assume no responsibility for your actions.

Any people depicted in stock imagery provided by Getty Images are models, and such images are being used for illustrative purposes only.
Certain stock imagery © Getty Images.

Print information available on the last page.

ISBN: 978-1-9822-8552-4 (sc)
ISBN: 978-1-9822-8553-1 (e)

Balboa Press rev. date: 06/20/2022

PART I

ESSENTIALS OF SURGICAL PRACTICE

PREFACE

The purpose of this booklet is to discuss some of the common problems a trainee is likely to confront when working in surgery. I believe it is important to get as much exposure as possible to various aspects of surgery when there is an opportunity to get it. Many of you may never have such an exposure in the future.

This compilation and arrangement of current knowledge is not a treatise; that is found elsewhere. Here, I have tried to go through topics as I would in a ward round. They are snippets. There are a number of illustrations to facilitate learning. Key information is highlighted.

The book is set in an easy-to-read format. *Snippets* has two volumes. Volume 1 deals with acute surgery and basic principles of perioperative care that underpin delivery of good care. Volume 2 deals with elective surgery.

This book will serve as a quick guide to managing surgical patients who are admitted acutely; it will also serve as a revision and give ideas for you to develop for the future. It can be used at foundation and core training levels. There are multiple choice questions at the end that will serve to embed your knowledge. Sadly, knowledge needs frequent recall before it embeds!

You will certainly need to read much more about these topics because this book only gives you snapshots of key aspects. I suggest that trainees enhance their knowledge and spend at least two hours a day reading around problems that they confront in day-to-day care of patients. One fact learnt well over a one day will give you 365 facts in a year! Information gained needs to be relearnt, assimilated, and implemented into practice.

Over time this knowledge will become the foundation for good practice, enabling better care of patients.

Nothing can supplant life skills learnt by simply being there and observing the management of surgical problems; watching how others confront problems over time will assist you in acquiring your own skills that will lead you to your goal.

I am always keen to state my own favourite quote: 'The attitude determines the altitude.' How high one flies is determined by one's attitude. This in turn is determined by your acquisition of competence, enthusiasm, compassion, humility, and ability to communicate.

Oscar Wilde said, 'You know more than you think you know, just as you know less than you want to know.'

Do take part in active discussions on the ward rounds and make the most of the period of training. Above all, enjoy the journey.

Best of luck.

Srinivasan Ravi
Consultant Surgeon

Blackpool, 2022

CONTENTS

THE SURGICALLY ILL PATIENT

The most important aspect of surgical clinical care is the ability to recognise and deal with the ill patients. The settings in which the patient presents to you will vary. In most cases, as a junior doctor, you are more likely to be confronted with ward patients than with outpatients. During the days when you are responsible for emergency admissions, there will be exposure to patients presenting acutely in the accident and emergency unit, critical care unit, or the wards. The locations in which one is called to review the patients may vary, but the criteria defining the degree of illness remain the same.

Patient care will often require support of senior colleagues. This may not always involve the surgical specialty alone and may include critical care, anaesthetics, and other medical and specialist surgical specialties.

Presentation of the Surgical Patient

There are three categories of presentation.

Acutely Ill. These patients need immediate resuscitation and action; they would have been rushed to the resuscitation area of the accident and emergency unit, or they may become ill in the wards during a period of observation and evaluation or from complications of procedures carried out in the hospital. They will need initiation of management concurrently with resuscitation and investigations.

1

Moderately Ill. These patients present with worsening problem over a few hours or days. In such cases, there will be time to take a proper history and then set out and process a plan of appropriate action.

Elective Patients. These patients are generally well, allowing time for routine investigation, assessment, and action.

The Acutely Ill Patient may need to be seen in the accident and emergency department or even in the resuscitation room, the acute surgical patient assessment unit, or the surgical wards due to worsening clinical condition. These patients may be unable to give any history and be in a state of collapse. They will need immediate resuscitation. In these situations, it is important to act expeditiously and in a planned and practiced manner.

Practice all the steps of the primary survey with colleagues and ensure fluency of approach that will stand you in good stead. It is also good to be aware of any ill patients in the wards at hand over so that you can be mentally prepared to act methodically.

The primary survey of ABCDE begins with the first principle.

I am sure you are all familiar with:

A:	Airway
B:	Breathing
C:	Circulation CVS
D:	Disability – CNS
E:	Exposure

Ensure that the patient's airway is patent and protected. This means that the patient is able to respond verbally. If there is no response, then ensure that the airway is made patent; this could be a simple step such as sweeping and suction of the oral cavity and ensuring that there is no collection or foreign body. There may be a need for insertion of an oropharyngeal tube such as the Guedel Airway. The next step in any acute surgical situation is to set up a high-flow oxygen mask with a reservoir and give sufficient oxygen to ensure maximum effect. This means the patient must have a pulse oximeter in place to monitor the oxygen saturation. This is often forgotten! Pulse oximeter measures oxygen saturation (SaO2).

There are many ways to give oxygen. The important message that cannot be overstated is that it should be given at the outset to all surgically ill patients. It is arguable that one should be cautious when dealing with a patient who has ongoing COPD. With monitoring, one can maximise the amount of oxygen that can be given safely because hypoxia is more likely to cause immediate problems.

Basics of Oxygen Delivery

Methods of delivery
- Nasal cannula
- Simple Mask
- Rebreathing Mask: permits admixture of inspired and expired air effectively increases dead space.
- Non-Rebreathing Mask: Oxygen flows through a reservoir to the mask. A valve prevents entry of exhaled air into the reservoir allowing a high concentration of oxygen to be delivered. This type of mask is used in hypoxic patients to deliver a high flow oxygen of 10-15 litres per minute under supervision
- Venturi Mask: Ideal for patients with COPD where the percentage of oxygen delivered must be constant. This mask is colour coded for flow rates from 24% to 60%.
- Laryngeal Mask
- Endotracheal intubation
- Tracheostomy

Terminology
Flow rate: the rate of flow of Oxygen can be increased or decreased by adjusting the flow from the oxygen tube.

FiO2: Fraction of inspired air. Normal air contains 21% oxygen The FiO2 for you and I therefore is 21%

PaO2: Partial pressure of oxygen in blood is 10-13.5kPa. (75-100 mmHg). Atmospheric pressure is 760mmHg. Oxygen being only 21% of the atmosphere generates a PARTIAL pressure of 21kPa or 160mmhg of a total atmospheric pressure. In the blood the PaO2 is lower than 21kPa because of shunting and admixture of dead space air with inspired air.

SaO2: Oxygen saturation as measured by the pulse oximeter. A saturation of 94% equates to a PaO2 of 8

Ensuring a good inflow of oxygen is just the first step. Delivery to the tissues, however, involves ensuring that there is enough fluid on board to carry the oxygen to where it is needed. The next step is to cannulate one or two veins and start optimising the blood volume with intravenous fluids. The type of fluid does not matter, but a good rule of thumb is 10–20 mL of crystalloid or colloid per kilogram body weight. In practice, in an 80–100 kg patient, it is about a litre of fluid. Most will need it. You may get it wrong occasionally, and the presentation may be that of an acute coronary event. It is therefore safe to give the fluid in aliquots of 200 mL stat with review and reassessment and, if needed, redirection of management. Another important point to note is that oxygen delivery is affected below a haemoglobin level of 80g/L (8 g/dL).

Sequentially or simultaneously, depending on the level of assistance available, the other steps of the primary survey must be put in place. Do not fail to check the blood sugar and, in a young woman, the pregnancy status!

Do not forget to call for help because a well-coordinated team is more likely to deliver good care!

Summary

- Talk to the patient and assess response
- Ensure airway is patent
- Set up high-flow oxygen if needed
- Put up a pulse oximeter and read it
- Cannulate and run in fluids 10–20 mL/kg
- Catheterise
- Check blood sugar; hypoglycaemia is often overlooked
- Call for assistance

Actions:

- Take a brief history from carers.
- Patients who are not stable need rapid action.

- Do not waste time. Call for immediate senior help.
- Start resuscitation procedure, which may need to go hand in hand with investigations.
- Avoid delays. Delays have a compounding effect.

Moderately ill patients are those who are able to talk to you and give a history. In these situations, you will have time to organise yourself to

- take a history and examine patient,
- make a plan of action and write it down,
- arrange investigations, and
- discuss with senior colleagues.

Elective patients are generally well. They would have been placed on an operation list for routine surgery. Up to 80 per cent of them may be day cases. They certainly will be able to give a history of their presenting complaint and may have had investigations carried out prior to admission. The investigations carried out previously must be reviewed at the time of admission. They may have comorbidity, which will need recognition and documentation. The medications, allergies, and particularly anticoagulants and the presence of diabetes must be noted.

Co-morbidity Evaluation
    Cardiac
    Respiratory
    Cerebro-vascular
    Renal
    Hepato-biliary
    Thrombo-embolic
    Metabolic – eg: diabetes
    Drugs – eg: anticoagulants/antiplatelets
    Dementia and lack of capacity

In summary, the assessment of the critically ill patients should follow a practiced protocol and should include the following.

- Primary assessment and immediate action as needed
- Review of all information that is available
- Secondary or reassessment
- Organisation of immediate investigations
- Plan of action based on the above
- Ongoing assessment followed by possible revision of the plan if needed
- Communication with seniors

Very often trainee doctors go through the various steps concentrating on the processes and failing to make the link between their observations and action. Look and link.

Act on abnormal observations. If an observation is abnormal, then it is abnormal. Do not find excuses to justify it but check it again and verify that it is truly abnormal. There is little point in making observations and then overlooking them.

When a patient is ill, attempt to get the physiology back in balance as soon as possible, if it is feasible. Recognise the following.

- Seriousness of a patient's illness
- Need to act expeditiously
- Predicting and preventing complications early saves lives
- Limitations of one's ability
- Benefits of consulting others
- Futility of a situation
- All life has a natural end
- Communication with surrogates (carers, family, next of kin) avoids conflict later

> **Rapid recognition of illness reduces complications** and will save lives.
>
> **Look, Link, Anticipate and Act** on abnormal findings early. Nip problems in the bud!

Many, but not all, ill patients will be in a state of systemic inflammatory response syndrome (SIRS). Illness tilts the physiological balance and manifests as SIRS in the early stages.

> **Systemic Inflammatory Response Syndrome**
>
> | | |
> |---|---|
> | T - Temperature | > 38.0 degrees C |
> | T - Tachycardia | > 90/min |
> | T - Tachypnoea | > 20/min |
> | T – Total white cell count | > 12 - < 4 |
>
> Note: Blood sugar may also be elevated in a non- diabetic. Mentation may be affected.
>
> If two of the above four are elevated the patient is deemed to be in a state of Systemic Inflammatory Response

Temperature is elevated because the hypothalamic thermostat is reset at a higher level due to elevated cytokines, especially interleukins.

Tachycardia occurs because the body needs to deliver more oxygen to the peripheries, and the patient may be fluid depleted. This is a sympathetic response.

Tachypnoea occurs when the patient is acidotic and tries to compensate by breathing out and eliminating carbon dioxide. Or the patient may be having abdominal pain, restricting breathing and manifesting as rapid, shallow breathing. Note that shallow breathing only moves the dead space air in and out of the bronchial tree and will not help oxygen delivery.

White cell response is characteristic of inflammation/infection and is mediated by interleukins. It is predominantly the neutrophil that leads this response when it is activated.

Activated neutrophil results in remote injury. Activation of the neutrophil is the key to the process of sepsis and is worth reading about in detail.

Three A's that lead the response	
Alarm	*the neutrophil raises the alarm*
Activation	*it rolls on endothelium diapedesis*
Amplification	*Mediates the cytokine response*

Here, you can see the movements of the activated neutrophil. On activation by a non-self antigen, the neutrophil becomes sticky. It crawls along the endothelium and then moves out of the vessel by diapedesis in the gaps between cells on to the area of inflammation. It then attacks the area of inflammation and attempts to kill the intruder. During this process, it undergoes lysis, and the process raises an alarm that initiates the complement and cytokine cascade. The neutrophil appears to call for help when needed!

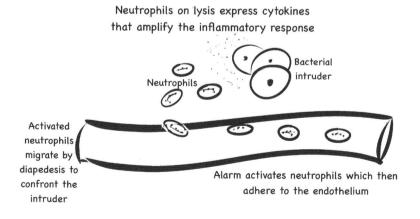

Figure 1: Activation and movement of neutrophil diapedesis.

The actual alarm cell is the dendritic cell, (originally noted by Ralph Steinman in 1973) found in the skin, gut and lungs in a less active form (immature) and in spleen in a more active form(mature). Immature dendritic cells promote phagocytosis – or **innate immunological response**. These cells populate an area of the body that is in contact with the outside world trying to stave off intrusion by **phagocytosis** or **'weep and sweep'** in the gut (producing mucus and diarrhoea). The mature cells set into action a more elaborate system referred to as the **adaptive immunity** by activating T cells to produce 'killer T cells and Helper T cells.

The phenomenal process of response to an intruder is outlined in great depth in the book, 'The Beautiful cure' (Feb 2018) by Daniel Davis.

The original work was started by Mechnikov in 1882, when he inserted thorns into star fish and noted the immediate movement of cells towards the thorn. Subsequently, these cells were named 'phagocyte' as it enveloped and killed bacteria. The larger cells when amalgamated in response to intrusion were named 'macrophage' or big killer!

Mechnikov also wrote a book on longevity. He held the view, that ageing is due to toxic gut organisms! In his book, he advocated the longevity of Bulgarians, to their yoghurt drink. He drank soured milk believing that the lactic acid due to lactobacillus was useful (LB Bulbaricum)

It is now appreciated that the systemic response that occurs with inflammation is an appropriate response to a focus of inflammation. In sepsis, the response that occurs is inappropriate and unregulated, setting off a cascade of physiological reactions that, if unrecognised early, lead to multiple systemic changes eventually leading to failure of organs and even death.

SEPSIS

The key feature of the syndrome of sepsis is the occurrence of manifestations remote from the site of insult. For example, cellulitis from a big toe infection in a diabetic can manifest as sepsis leading to multi-organ failure. At the site, it manifests as infection and cellulitis, but systemically it can manifest as full-blown sepsis.

Remote tissues show the effects of

- inflammation,
- vasodilatation,
- increased vascular permeability, and
- leucocyte accumulation.

It is a cogwheel in which the processes of sepsis are intertwined. It starts with physiological disruption and decrease in oxygen being delivered to the tissues. The oxygen deficit leads to mediator activation. The mediators are many, varied, and determined by multiple factors, including response to the insult being genetically different for different individuals. Some patients with severe sepsis may recover after ITU care whilst some with minimal sepsis may succumb. The response to treatment is unpredictable.

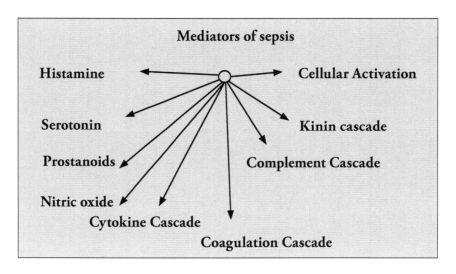

Once this process is entrenched, the changes can become difficult to control, much as a juggler taking on more and more balls finds it difficult to keep all balls in play and inevitably fails. The progressive failure to regain physiological control leads to multi-organ failure and then to death.

The process starts with oxygen debt. Sepsis follows on from potentiating events of cell injury secondary to oxygen debt that is often remote from the primary site of origin.

There is a massive and uncontrolled release of pro-inflammatory mediators such as interleukin 6 and other cytokines. This is called the cytokine storm. The chain of events becomes uncontrolled, unregulated, and self-sustaining.

Potentiating effect of multiple cell injury

Initially the cell injury causes **hypoxia**.

Hypoxia, then leads to further cell injury.

On reperfusion with fluids and correction of hypoxia, the reperfusion injury in itself, leads to further cell injury.

The cell injury then once more leads to inability to use oxygen and to **oxygen debt**.

Oxygen debt initiates **mediator response** of sepsis and the process gets out of control.

That leads to **multiple organ failure**.

Multiple organ failure can lead to **death**.

It is necessary, therefore, to ensure the level of oxygen in the air that is breathed in is optimised. The tissue utilisation of available oxygen is a matter of the pathophysiology that drives sepsis and may be difficult to control. Ensuring that the inspired air contains sufficient oxygen that can be delivered to the tissue is the reason for the insistence that in surgically ill patients, the first step in management is to maximise the inspired oxygen by setting up high flow oxygen by mask and giving intravenous fluids to ensure that the oxygen can be delivered to the tissues. Checking the oxygen saturation and blood pressure are thus the first steps in resuscitation.

Houtchens BA, Westenskow DR. Oxygen consumption in septic shock: collective review. Circ Shock. 1984;13(4):361-84.

That a decline in oxygen consumption (VO2) might herald onset of septic shock prior to hemodynamic collapse is suggested by previous observations in humans and animals in which VO2 appeared to be suppressed in systemic sepsis, despite normal or supranormal cardiac output, and in cellular and mitochondrial preparations exposed to endotoxin, despite adequate flow of perfusate. That a supranormal VO2 might be one of the best predictors of ultimate survival is suggested by data collected from humans during various stages of septic shock.

Timely prediction of possible progress and rapid remedial actions at the early stages may break the cog wheel and the chain of self-sustaining progression towards multiple organ failure and inevitable death.

Early recognition of sepsis is possible with monitoring of respiratory rate, drop in blood pressure, and changes in mentation. This is the basis of qSOFA (quick Sequential Organ Failure Assessment), a method for early appreciation of sepsis. If two of the three parameters are abnormal, the patient should be screened for sepsis. The SOFA scoring system is laborious and difficult to implement without reference to it. However, the qSOFA is easy, and recognition of abnormality should raise suspicion that the patient may be harbouring a focus of sepsis.

---

qSOFA
quick Sequential Organ Failure Assessment
Bed side assessment

1. Tachypnoea: greater than 22
2. Hypotension systolic less than 100 mmhg
3. Altered Mentation – GCS less than 15

Each is awarded one point. 2 points indicates an increased possibility of sepsis in non ITU patients.

Look, Link, Anticipate, Act

Once sepsis is suspected, it must be excluded by using the 'sepsis six'.

Sepsis six

1. Administer Oxygen to maintain saturation > 94%
2. Take blood cultures at least a peripheral set. Think source control – may need CSF/Urine/sputum cultures
3. Give Intravenous antibiotics as per protocol within the hour
4. Administer Intravenous fluids at 10-20 ml/kg initially
5. Check serum lactate levels
6. Measure urine output

Give 3/Take 3!
Give Oxygen/fluids/antibiotics
Take cultures/serum lactate/urine sample

Management of critically ill surgical patients must occur on the threshold of the operating theatre. It is best done in collaboration with the critical care team because the situation may progress rapidly to the patient, requiring higher and higher levels of care. Knowing the principles of care enables erudite discussion with colleagues.

Singer M, Deutschman CS, Seymour CW, et al. **The Third International Consensus Definitions for Sepsis and Septic Shock** (Sepsis-3). *JAMA.* 2016;315(8):801–810.

Key Findings from Evidence Synthesis- Limitations of previous definitions included an excessive focus on inflammation, the misleading model that sepsis follows a continuum through severe sepsis to shock, and inadequate specificity and sensitivity of the systemic inflammatory response syndrome (SIRS) criteria. Multiple definitions and terminologies are currently in use for sepsis, septic shock, and organ dysfunction, leading to discrepancies in reported incidence and observed mortality. The task force concluded the term *severe sepsis* was redundant.

Recommendations: Sepsis should be defined as life-threatening organ dysfunction caused by a dysregulated host response to infection. For clinical operationalization, organ dysfunction can be represented by an increase in the Sequential [Sepsis-related] Organ Failure Assessment (SOFA) score of 2 points or more, which is associated with an **in-hospital mortality greater than 10%.** Septic shock should be defined as a subset of sepsis in which particularly profound circulatory, cellular, and metabolic abnormalities are associated with a greater risk of mortality than with sepsis alone. Patients with septic shock can be clinically identified by a vasopressor requirement to maintain **a mean arterial pressure of 65 mm Hg** or greater and **serum lactate level greater than 2 mmol/L (>18 mg/dL) in the absence of hypovolemia**. This combination is associated with **hospital mortality rates greater than 40%.** In out-of-hospital, emergency department, or general hospital ward settings, adult patients with suspected infection can be rapidly identified as being more likely to have poor outcomes typical of sepsis if they have at least 2 of the following clinical criteria that together constitute **a new bedside clinical score termed quickSOFA (qSOFA): respiratory rate of 22/min or greater, altered mentation, or systolic blood pressure of 100 mm Hg or less.**

Conclusions and Relevance These updated definitions and clinical criteria should replace previous definitions, offer greater consistency for epidemiologic studies and clinical trials, and facilitate earlier recognition and more timely management of patients with sepsis or at risk of developing sepsis.

Therapeutic Priorities

Counter physiologic abnormalities and attempt to bring them back to normal if possible. Every organism needs the same basic requirements for survival: air, water, food, and shelter. Mitigate the effects of loss by attention to these factors as follows:

- Air (hypoxemia)— **Deliver oxygen**
- Water (hypotension)— **Give fluids**
- Food—**Nutrition**
- Shelter—**ITU, HDU**

Goals of therapy for initial resuscitation are universal.

- Replete circulation
- Identify source of loss
- Prevent further loss
- Replete loss

Distinguishing Sepsis from SIRS can be useful. As stated earlier, the inflammatory response to insult could be an appropriate or an inappropriate response. If a patient is in a state of systemic inflammatory response, then greater attention must be paid to the patient, and the reason for the response must be evaluated.

Identify and treat the source of infection. It is all too easy to discharge a patient with abdominal discomfort, a high white cell count, and a tachycardia only to find later that the patient had a perforated diverticulum of the sigmoid. Valuable time can thus be lost. Look and link the abnormality to the clinical findings.

- **Cultures**—Blood, urine, sputum (**BUS**)
- **Radiology**—CXR, CT scan, USS, MRI
- **Interventions**—Drainage of focus radiologically/surgically
- **Antibiotics**—Discuss with microbiologists the appropriate antibiotics needed for a particular situation

Principles of management are the same for all surgical emergencies.

Principles of Management

Immediate assessment: ABCDE
> Never forget pulse oximetry

Immediate investigations:
> **Urine** for nitrates, beta-hcg, sugar and blood
>
> **Blood** for sugar, full blood count, electrolytes and urea, coagulation profile
>
> **Radiology** for assisting assessment and diagnosis including erect chest x-ray, USS and CT scan

Comorbidity assessment such as ECG to exclude acute myocardial event, diabetes, COPD, renal status and anti-coagulants

Call for Assistance/Allied speciality advice

The SILDA Mantra

Stabilisation: Blood pressure over 90mmhg/O2 >94%

Investigation: Concurrently with making the patient stable

Localisation: Find the cause

Decision: Type of care- conservative, interventional, palliative

Action: Prompt action saves lives. No vacillation

The following is reproduced from NICE guidance on critical care.

The national early warning score (NEWS) is based on a simple aggregate scoring system in which a score is allocated to physiological measurements, already recorded in routine practice, when patients present to or are being monitored in hospital.

Six simple physiological parameters form the basis of the scoring system.

- Respiration rate
- Oxygen saturation
- Systolic blood pressure
- Pulse rate

- Level of consciousness or new confusion[1]
- Temperature.

The score is then aggregated and uplifted by 2 points for people requiring supplemental oxygen to maintain their recommended oxygen saturation.

Physiological Parameter	3	2	1	0	1	2	3
Respiration rate/min	≤ 8		9–11	**12–20**		21–24	≥ 25
S_pO^2 (Normal)%	≤ 91	92-93	93–94	**≥ 96**			
S_pO^2 (COPD)%	≤83	84–85	86–87	**88–92** **≥ 93**	93–94 oxygen	95–96 oxygen	≥ 97 oxygen
Systolic Blood pressure(mmHg)	≤ 90	91–100	101–110	**111–219**			≥ 220
Pulse rate	≤ 40		41–50	**51–90**	91–110	111–130	≥ 131
Consciousness				**alert**			CVPU
Temperature (°C)	≤ 35		35.1–36.0	**36.1–38.0**	38.1–39.0	> 39.1	

The NEWS is based on Royal College of Physicians working party (2017). Note that oxygen delivery adds 2 to the score. A score of 0, 1, 2, or 3 is allocated to each parameter. A higher score means the parameter is further out from the normal range.

The score is used to trigger appropriate response. This is the basis of track and trigger. The trigger levels are nationally formulated but must be locally agreed and implemented.

> **Low risk** (aggregate score 1–4)—prompt assessment by ward nurse to decide on change to frequency of monitoring or escalation of clinical care

> **Low to medium risk** (score of 3 in any single parameter)—urgent review by ward-based team of nurses or doctors to determine cause

---

[1] Where previously their mental state was normal, any new mental change may be subtle. The patient may respond to questions coherently, but there may be confusion, disorientation, and/or agitation. This would score 3 or 4 on the GCS (rather than the normal 5 for verbal response), and it scores 3 on the NEWS system.

and decide on change to frequency of monitoring or escalation of clinical care

Medium risk (aggregate score 5–6)—urgent review by ward-based doctor or acute team nurse to decide on escalation to critical care team

High risk (aggregate score of 7 or higher)—emergency assessment by critical care team, usually leading to patient transfer to higher-dependency care area

Levels of Care

- Level 0 care is care in the normal wards
- Level 1 care is care in a specialist acute ward such as a post-operative ward
- Level 2 care is high dependency unit (HDU) care, where there is a need to support one major organ system.
- Level 3 care is intensive care unit (ICU) level care, when there is a need to support two organ systems and/or respiratory support.

WHO Performance Status

- **0**: Can carry out normal activity without restriction
- **1**: Restricted in strenuous activity; can carry out light work
- **2**: Capable of all self-care; unable to carry out any work activities; up and about more than 50 per cent of waking hours
- **3**: Symptomatic and in a chair or in bed for greater than 50 per cent of the day, but not bedridden
- **4**: Completely disabled; cannot carry out any self-care; totally confined to bed or chair

Increasingly, the performance status of a patient is being taken into consideration prior to major interventions that may not be of benefit to the patient.

The Early warning scoring system is a familiar concept. The principle behind it has been noted by many practitioners of medicine in the past in one form or another. Pertaining to surgical practice, a form of this concept was pioneered by Ochsner-Sherren in the early 20th century.

It's application in the treatment of acute appendicitis was commented on by **Hamilton Bailey in a BMJ article in 1930.** He believed, that with respect to appendicitis the concept of waiting, monitoring and watching had a role.

The principle was to monitor the pulse rate, the temperature and the size of the appendicular mass. As long as they seemed to be improving, there was no need for immediate surgical operative intervention. If the parameters worsened, then it was necessary to operate on an appendicular mass. Mind you, those were the days prior to the advent of antibiotics. Peritonitis meant death. Abscesses were drained extra peritoneally as intraperitoneal contamination meant certain death.

Hamilton Bailey added that the 'observation policy' was applicable when patients presented 'Too late for the early operation and too early for the late operation.

He cautioned, that the policy of observation should not be at the cost of consideration of a timely operation saying that 'Evil lies in the abuse of all good things'

This paper is available on line for those interested in the evolution of aspects of surgical care.

ETHICS

Management of any patient must be tempered with compassion and empathy. It is best to try to imagine yourself in the position of the patient and their family. It must be remembered that all autonomy is lost when a patient is admitted to the hospital for acute care. This transformation is immediate, and the role of the treating physician becomes one of authority. This position must be upheld with care and concern. The first principle is *primum non nocere*, which translates to 'First do no harm'. To this, one can add 'Do the best you can.' Always.

The following are factors that need consideration.

- Loss of autonomy
- Withholding or withdrawing treatment
- Futility and frailty
- Consent and capacity
- Combined decision-making
- Deviation from the norm

Loss of Autonomy

This is quite difficult to understand, but as one gains experience, the work will teach you. When working in a place of authority, the position confers a degree of authority to the treating healthcare workers. Many patients find it difficult to challenge authority even if its recommendations differ from their wishes. It is worthwhile going through the Stanley Milgram experiments on obedience. When position confers authority, it necessary to use it with care. Many patients will agree to most things if they like the treating doctor, and they will try to oblige by giving the answers that the doctor expects rather than disagree. Very often, discussions with surrogates and next of kin may help in divining what the patient really wants.

Stanley Milgram's Experiments with Obedience

Stanley Milgram a Psychologist working in Yale University in the early 1960's was curious about how a whole nation such as Germany blindly followed the Nazi ideals. He devised an experiment in which he advised random public participants to give increasing levels of fake 'electric shock' to 'learners'. The participants were informed that this experiment was being conducted under the authority of the Government of the United States. The fake electric shocks were increased to fatal levels and when participants questioned it as it was against their conscience, they were prompted to carry on administering increasing levels of shock because this study was approved by a higher authority. Not all did so, but most carried out the written guidance to the full without questioning it. This experiment was discredited subsequently on the basis of 'research ethics' but more than 80% of the participants were glad to have participated. The results of the experiment suggests that in principle people will follow authority without questioning it. It is therefore necessary to use the position of authority with care.

GMC Guidance: Withholding and Withdrawing Treatment

This is a must-read for all. The document is available online. This is an excerpt from the original.

- Doctors have a responsibility to make the care of their patients their first concern. This is essential when considering any of the growing range of life-prolonging treatments which make it possible to extend the lives of patients who, through organ failure or other life-threatening conditions, might otherwise die.

- The benefits of modern techniques such as cardiopulmonary resuscitation, renal dialysis, artificial ventilation, and artificial nutrition and hydration, are considerable. However, life has a natural end, and the existence of such techniques presents doctors, patients and their families with dilemmas.
- Dilemmas arise where, for example, advanced techniques of life support may be able, in some cases where patients are in a permanent vegetative state or similar condition, to sustain life artificially for many years with little or no hope of recovery. In other cases, they may simply prolong the dying process and cause unnecessary distress to the patient.
- In these instances, the question arises as to whether it is in the best interests of the patient to start or continue the treatment. Reaching a satisfactory answer may mean addressing a number of difficult ethical and legal issues.

The main questions that arise are as follows.

- Would the ethical principle requiring doctors to show respect for human life mean that doctors should offer all means at their disposal to prolong a patient's life? Or would it allow for the possibility of withholding or withdrawing life-prolonging treatment that would be unlawful?
- What are the responsibilities in the decision-making process of the patient, doctor, healthcare team, family members, and other people who are close to the patient? And what weight should be given to their views?

These issues have caused considerable debate amongst the profession and the public, and in the courts, highlighting a number of concerns within the wider community. These include concerns about the following.

- The possibility of over- or under-treatment towards the end of life

- Concerns that some doctors may make decisions about life-prolonging treatments without access to up-to-date clinical advice
- Concerns that doctors may make judgements about the appropriateness of treatment (or non-treatment) on a quality-of-life basis regarding patients, particularly the very young or very old, which patients or society as a whole may not support

It is also clear that the profession and patients want more guidance on what is considered ethically and legally permissible in this area, and that patient and their families want greater involvement in making these decisions, with better arrangements to support them when facing these distressing situations.

Futility and Frailty

Futility can be classified as follows.

- Physiological futility
- Anatomical futility
- Social futility

In physiological futility, possibility of imminent death is included. An old surgical adage, now implemented with political awareness, is that, 'If a patient is dying imminently or recovering rapidly, do not intervene.' Nature may be allowed to take its course, for instance after a second cardiac arrest on the ward after a failed resuscitation. Seldom if ever do patients survive a second cardiac arrest. Physiological futility is a surgical situation where the GCS is less than 5, and there may be little point in attempting heroic interventions. There are always exceptions to all rules, and that must also be borne in mind.

Anatomical futility is a situation when, after a road traffic accident, the body is so badly mangled that it cannot be meaningfully reconstructed.

Social futility is difficult to judge. There are situations when a patient cannot be returned to the same lifestyle as the patient was used to prior to admission to the hospital for treatment. Take for example an elderly patient with dementia who presents with a colonic perforation. It is likely that the carer is an equally elderly partner. In these situations, it is more than likely that following the operation, the dementia may worsen, leading to inability for the carer to look after the patient at home. The patient may then need to be admitted to a nursing home with major implications for the future. These situations merit discussions with the next of kin and will require a best interest meeting to assist the decision making process. In times of emergency, the latter may not be feasible, and it may be best to be guided by surrogates. Consenting for surgery, however, will also require a best interest meeting.

Frailty

The ageing process takes its toll, and unfortunately there is no return to a better state of health that is possible for most. (Nortin Hadler) Frailty is a recognised factor that increases morbidity and mortality after any type of surgery.

A quick rule of thumb for assessing frailty is the following.

- Hand grip strength
- Sitting to standing time
- Walking speed

Rockwood Clinical Frailty Score

1. Very Fit: Exercise regularly/robust
2. Well: Exercise occasionally/no active symptoms
3. Managing Well: Controlled medical problems
4. Vulnerable: Symptoms limit activities/independence
5. Mildly Frail: Slow with inside and outside activities
6. Moderately Frail: Help with all outside activities
7. Severely Frail: Full dependence for personal care
8. Very Severely Frail: Approaching end of life

Rockwood Score in Dementia

1. Mild: Forgetting recent events; repeating stories and questions
2. Moderate: Recent memory very impaired; attend to personal care with prompting; recall past events well
3. Severe: Cannot do personal care without help

Capacity and Consenting

Capacity is the cognitive function that allows us to take in new information, retain that information, and weigh the pros and cons of that information prior to coming to a decision about whether the information is in keeping with one's judgement.

Capacity is not binary; it is a spectrum, and the grey area may involve assisted decision-making or co-decision-making, with legal implications. Capacity cannot be taken for granted in the ill patients because it is quite likely that illness itself has taken away capacity. It must be borne in mind that the loss of capacity may be transient due to an illness such as sepsis, or it may be an established loss due to dementia or other illness. It is always necessary to assess capacity, and if a patient is thought not to have capacity to make a judgement, then one must involve the family or surrogates in the decision-making process. It may be necessary to call for a best interest meeting with surrogates to decide on the most acceptable modality of treatment, which may include non-treatment. Capacity merits careful consideration along with frailty and dementia. It may be acceptable in certain situations to agree to a surgical intervention for a time-limited period, defer the final decision for a period of forty-eight hours after surgical intervention, and then convene a meeting to make a final decision depending on the progress that has been made by the patient. Consultation with anaesthetists or a critical care team in these situations is invaluable. Avoiding conflict with the family and carers is pre-eminent.

Consent to intervention of any sort forms part of the same discussion. Some patients may already have considered aspects of end of life and decided on levels of care that they would like implemented. This may be presented as an **advance directive**. An advance directive is a legal document that clearly outlines the wishes of the patient about future medical care. It may state the level of care that the patient would like implemented including, 'Do Not Attempt Resuscitation' **(DNAR)** orders. As it is a legal document, the stated wishes of the patient must be implemented.

The principles of decision making are as follows.

- Disease related
- Patient related
- Technique related

It is important to reflect on the fact that the feasibility of an operation is not an indication for its performance. Every patient must be assessed from the point of futility and risk of mortality and morbidity for any operation. The assessment is required for both elective and emergency surgery. In the elective situations, the decision to operate may be assisted, and in some patients corrected, by pre-operative interventions; these include discussing weight loss in the obese and respiratory function in patients with COPD, or operating in summer rather than winter.

Breaking Bad News

This is best done by doctors with experience and knowledge of the situation. Whilst bad news is not always life-threatening, it changes the future for the patient, family, friends, and relatives. The manner of communication must be considered, genuine, and well meaning. Bad news is unpleasant, and the behaviour of the informant must reflect the seriousness of the situation with due preparation and planning about the manner of information delivery and inclusion of appropriate staff members.

Practical Principles

Ensure that the patient is reviewed daily.

Consider the care of the patient as a contract between the two individuals, carer and cared. Deal with every patient as one would like to be dealt with oneself. Apply these principles universally.

When King Edward VII was being treated for cor pulmonale by Bertie Dawson of the London hospital he asked how he proposed treating him. 'Sire' replied Dawson 'I shall treat you like any of my patients in the wards at the London Hospital'.

Treatment of patients should be guided by standard principles because any deviation from the norm can lead to disaster.

General Principles of Clinical Examination

First principles

- Make the connection
- Introduce yourself
- Verify and confirm demographics
- Explain why you are there
- Seek permission to examine
- Wash your hands
- Ask if there is any area of pain or tenderness
- Be gentle and reassuring

Abdomen

- Inspect from the foot end of bed or side.
- Ask the patient to cough; look for any cough impulse.
- Note location of umbilicus, presence of scars/lumps/veins/other abnormalities.
- Palpate away from the site of pain, if any. If there is no area of pain, then from the left lower quadrant upwards and around in an anticlockwise manner. It is best not to dig with one's fingers but feel with the flat of the hand. If there is a palpable mass, then note if it moves with respiration or if it is fixed.
- For hernia, examine the patient standing up and confirm the presence of the hernia. Lie the patient down and gently compress the internal ring region, roughly, a couple of fingers above the middle of the inguinal ligament. Ask the patient to cough while compressing and inspecting the groin. If it is a direct hernia, the lump will reappear despite the compression of the internal ring. An indirect hernia will be contained by compression.

Even though current fashion is to proceed to radiology assisted diagnosis with a CT scan or an ultrasound, it is a good principle to examine the patient clinically as it creates a rapport which, if gentle, will go a long way towards reassuring the patient whose illness would have taken away his autonomy.

THE ACUTE ABDOMEN

There is no simple definition of an acute abdomen other than to say that it is a combination of signs and symptoms that necessitate referral for urgent general surgical opinion. Making a diagnosis is an imprecise art. It taxes the skills of experienced surgeons and requires pragmatism. The classic presentations commonly described are not seen commonly. There is a greater dependence on radiological colleagues to assist the diagnostic process. Even so, very often time and monitoring with repeated reviews of the patient will aid delivery of good care. The most important decision may not always be the diagnosis but the decision to operate or withhold operation. If a decision is made to operate, then the next decision is the consideration of the timing of the operation. Should the operation be done immediately or can it wait till suitable arrangements and resuscitation can be achieved. As noted previously evaluation of the morbidity and mortality and involvement of appropriate surrogates in the decision-making process is mandatory.

The common surgical problems that one confronts during surgical practice can be divided into two groups.

- Problems that arise from the acute presentation with abdominal pain that need immediate treatment
- Problems that arise that need to be treated on a non-acute basis

In the acute surgical setting the management involves, recognition of the presentation and defining the immediate management. A decision must be taken to prioritise the surgical treatment as

- Immediate
- Early (within twenty-four to forty-eight hours)
- Elective (where resolution of urgent problem permits a scheduled treatment)

Certain points are worth clarifying:

- It is noteworthy that management is not always only surgical.
- The feasibility of an operation is not an indication for its performance.
- Futility of a situation due to comorbidity is part of the decision-making process.
- If an emergency operation is needed and the patient fit for surgery, procrastination is detrimental to successful outcome.
- If the patient is unsuitable for intervention, it must be discussed with the patient and family and documented.
- If a decision is taken that further care will not be in the best interest of the patient, a Do Not Attempt Resuscitation (DNAR) form needs to be completed.

Abdominal zones

The abdomen is classically divided into nine zones for ease of description. It defines zones that are related to underlying structures. From the surgical viewpoint as opposed to the classical, we have four quadrants. Interestingly, if we name them according to the common presenting problems in each quadrant, then the quadrants are respectively, biliary, appendicular, splenic, and diverticular.

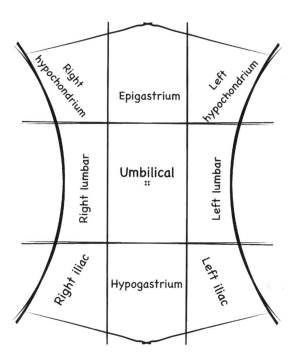

Figure 2: Classical abdominal zones

This simplified version does not explain all the possibilities but only directs the thinking process to the common probabilities of presenting problems.

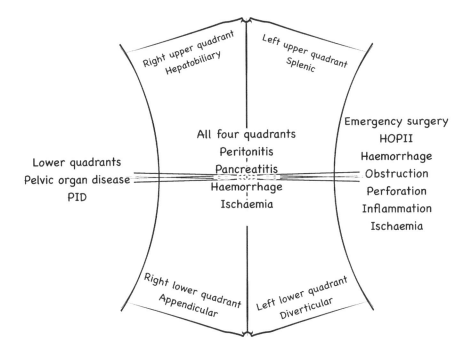

Figure 3: Practical abdominal zones

When there is a presentation involving all four quadrants, peritonitis, pancreatitis, and vascular emergencies must be considered. Peritonitis is generally a four-quadrant disease but can be localised to a quadrant when pathological process is contained by the process of nature.

RUQ	Cholecystitis, biliary colic, hepatitis, duodenal ulcer
Epigastrium	Peptic ulcer disease, oesophagitis, pancreatitis, myocardial infarction
RLQ	Appendicitis, PID, Crohn's, urinary infections/calculi, Right colon carcinoma, Meckel's
LUQ	Splenic pathology, pancreatitis
LLQ	Diverticulitis, PID, urinary infections/calculi, recto sigmoid carcinoma

An important surface marking is the transpyloric plane. If you can visualise the structures in this plane, you can appreciate the probable pathologies that can arise. It must always be borne in mind that autonomic pain can be difficult to localise unlike somatic pain.

The Trans-pyloric plane extends between the ninth ribs and bisects the upper abdomen. Located in it are the following:

- Fundus of the gall bladder
- Pylorus of the stomach
- Origin of SMA
- Hilum of the spleen
- Second part of duodenum
- Neck of pancreas
- Hila of the kidneys
- Origin of portal vein

PERITONITIS

The peritoneum is a cling-film-like serous layer that sticks to the viscera and to the inner wall of the abdominal cavity much like an invaginated balloon. It has a visceral and a parietal layer.

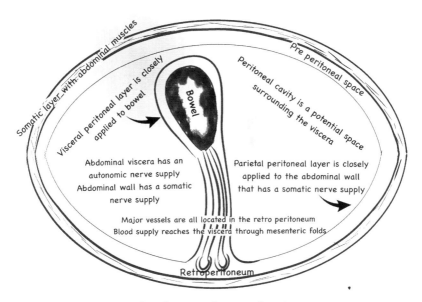

Figure 4: Schematic layout of peritoneum

The peritoneal cavity is a potential space unlike this stylised diagram. The loops of bowel are normally in contact with the abdominal wall, and to facilitate movement without friction, there is a thin sliver of peritoneal fluid that acts as a lubricant. Mesentery is the structure lined by peritoneum that allows the transmission of blood vessels from the retroperitoneum to the viscera. It is worthy of note that the kidneys and pancreas are behind the peritoneum, or in the retroperitoneum.

When there is perforation of viscus or when there is inflammation of the pancreas there is fluid extrusion; the peritoneum gets inflamed and leads to peritonitis. Peritonitis can be chemical or bacterial. When peritonitis occurs, there is excess accumulation of fluid within the peritoneal cavity due to a combination of secretion and/or extrusion of intraluminal contents. The initial response is to a chemical irritation, but after six to twelve hours, a bacterial overgrowth sets in. This is the reason for the need for early action rather than waiting till the next morning for convenience. Timely action saves lives.

The fluid then collects in two areas of the peritoneal cavity that are most dependent in the supine posture: the pelvis, and the Rutherford Morrison pouch, which is between the liver and the kidney. This is therefore, the reason why abscesses commonly tend to occur in the pelvis, and sub-hepatic areas of the peritoneal cavity.

Peritoneal fluid can also arise from non-inflammatory causes such as in malignancy and cirrhosis of the liver. When there is an increase in peritoneal fluid alone without any inflammation, it is called ascites.

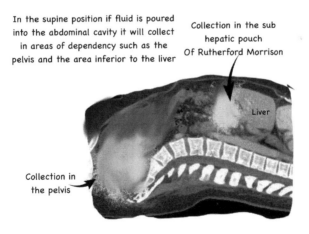

In the supine position if fluid is poured into the abdominal cavity it will collect in areas of dependency such as the pelvis and the area inferior to the liver

Collection in the sub hepatic pouch Of Rutherford Morrison

Liver

Collection in the pelvis

In the days before modern imaging, in patients with sepsis, the surgical adage was " pus some where, pus no where, pus under the diaphragm". Now a days, imaging defines intra abdominal collections. The new adage should be " sepsis somewhere, sepsis no where, sepsis in the central lines"

Figure 5: Pelvic collection in dependent areas

When the peritoneal fluid is collection is due to a leakage from blood vessels, it is referred to as haemorrhagic ascites.

Causes of Peritonitis

- Perforated viscus due to:
  - Peptic perforation
  - Appendicular perforation
  - Colonic-diverticular perforation
  - Gall bladder perforation
  - Small bowel perforation
  - Meckel's perforation
  - Malignant bowel perforation
  - Anastomotic leak
- Ectopic pregnancy
- Ruptured aneurysm of abdominal aorta
- Tubo-ovarian abscess
- Penetrating injury
- Ischaemic bowel
- Pancreatitis

Presenting Symptoms and Signs

- Pain is the major presenting symptom. It is stated that peritonitis due to perforation of peptic ulcer, pancreatitis, ischaemia, and ruptured abdominal aortic aneurysms are the most severe.
- Nausea may precede pain and vomiting usually follows.
- Tachypnoea occurs due to pain and acidosis.
- Tachycardia.
- Altered mentation.

Abdominal Findings on Examination

Tenderness, generalised. As opposed to localised tenderness, when there is an attempt to contain the pathological process.

Rebound tenderness. This is a classical finding when there is pain on pressure and pain on release of pressure on the abdominal wall. The less intrusive way of demonstrating this is to do a gentle percussion. If the percussion causes pain, then rebound tenderness is most likely to be present.

Guarding. This is a protective response to pain when the muscles overlying the pathology contract and tighten to protect the viscera by stiffening to the threat of being pushed.

Rigidity. The abdomen is board like and tense due to all the abdominal muscles contracting and stiffening. This is a protective response like guarding and attempts to reduce movements that cause pain.

The management then follows the principles laid out in the earlier chapter.

PEPTIC PERFORATION

This used to be a very common surgical emergency. The advent of H_2 receptor blockade with cimetidine in the late seventies and subsequent identification of Helicobacter pylori **(H. pylori)** as the causative factor for peptic ulcer has made this disease increasingly less common. Prior to Marshall's identification of the causative organism for most peptic ulcers, the treatment of peptic disease was mostly surgical. Now it is mostly medical.

Peptic ulcers arise in areas of the gastrointestinal tree that are exposed to acid peptic digestion. The key here is that there must be a combination of both acid and pepsin. The pepsin, which digests proteins, is made from the precursor, pepsinogen. The acid in the stomach cleaves the pepsinogen to pepsin and makes it active. The areas that are exposed to it are the lower oesophagus, stomach, and duodenum but also the Meckel's diverticulum, which may have ectopic gastric cells. It follows that areas exposed to peptic digestion may also suffer peptic perforation and bleeding. Peptic bleeding can still occur due to the usage of aspirin and non-steroidals, but they can almost all be managed endoscopically.

Patients presenting with duodenal ulcers are nearly all infected with H. pylori (90 per cent). Marshall says, 'It is very unlikely that persons without H. pylori infections will ever develop duodenal ulcer.'

Gastric ulcers are also caused by H. pylori, but up to about 30 per cent may be related to treatment with aspirin or non-steroidals. It is good practice to treat all patients presenting with peptic ulcer perforation as being infected with H. pylori by giving them the appropriate antibiotic treatment along with high-dose proton pump inhibitor. The treatment must be for a period of no fewer than ten days and possibly for fourteen days.

Antibiotic treatment for H. pylori eradication following perforated peptic disease is best initiated prior to discharge from hospital after surgery. The treatment that is recommended for peptic disease in dyspeptic patients after confirmation of H. pylori infection with a urea breath test is also applicable following perforated peptic disease.

The recommended first-line treatment for H. pylori is for seven days.

- PPI twice daily
- Amoxicillin 1g BD

Plus

- Clarithromycin 500mg BD

Or

- Metronidazole 400mg BD

If allergic to penicillin, Clarithromycin and metronidazole can be prescribed.

The protocol may vary in different countries. Successful eradication of H. pylori must be confirmed with a urea breath test on completion of the course. In the United States, the recommended treatment is for fourteen days.

Presentation of Peptic Perforation

As with all peritonitis, the signs may be localized or generalised. Classically, the abdomen is rigid like a board, and the patient is in severe pain with possibly altered mentation, tachycardia, and tachypnoea. The initial pain for the first six hours is likely to be due to chemical peritonitis caused by spillage of gastro-duodenal contents. This is rapidly followed by the onset of bacterial peritonitis within twelve hours, stressing the need for rapid intervention in the suitable patients rather than waiting and watching.

The erect chest X-ray showing free gas may not be possible if the patient is in severe pain. A semi-erect X-ray with the patient sitting up in bed may help define the presence of free air under the diaphragm. A CT scan is quick and gives you the same information, obviating the need to repeat investigations. Air under the diaphragm is due to free air and not air that is contained within the bowel. The Chilaiditi sign, due to an entrapped loop of hepatic flexure between the diaphragm and liver, may mimic free gas under the diaphragm, but these are rare signs, and the gas is always within the lumen of the bowel. Free gas of perforated viscus lies out side the lumen of the stomach and bowel and can be located under the hemidiaphragms.

The principles of management are substantially the same for all patients presenting with peritonitis.

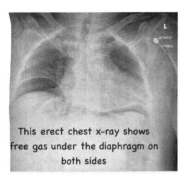

This erect chest x-ray shows free gas under the diaphragm on both sides

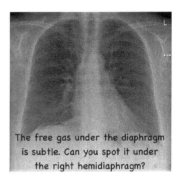

The free gas under the diaphragm is subtle. Can you spot it under the right hemidiaphragm?

The presence of free gas under the diaphragm indicates perforation of intraperitoneal viscus such as stomach or colon. Occasionally, the free gas may be retroperitoneal as with perforations of the posterior wall of the duodenum. These are difficult to recognise on an erect chest x-ray

Figure 6 Erect x-ray of the chest showing free gas

As stated earlier, these assessments should be done on the threshold of the operating theatre. Assessment, resuscitation, and anaesthetic advice must all go hand in hand. Not all patients will be suitable for surgical intervention. Assessment of fitness, morbidity, and mortality from surgical intervention must be made in conjunction with an anaesthetist.

Principles of Management

Immediate assessment: ABCDE
> Never forget pulse oximetry

Immediate investigations:
> **Urine** for nitrates, beta-hcg, sugar and blood
> Blood for sugar, full blood count, electrolytes and urea, coagulation profile
> Radiology for assisting assessment and diagnosis including erect chest x-ray, USS and CT scan

Comorbidity assessment such as ECG to exclude acute myocardial event, diabetes, COPD, renal status and anti-coagulants

Call for Assistance/Allied speciality advice

If sepsis is suspected, follow sepsis six protocol – this means giving timely antibiotics and fluid pending interventional management.

The SILDA Mantra

Stabilisation: Blood pressure over 90mmhg/O2 >94%
Investigation: Concurrently with making the patient stable
Localisation: Find the cause
Decision: Type of care- conservative, interventional, palliative
Action: Prompt action saves lives. No vacillation

The principle that should not be overlooked is, 'Feasibility of an operation is not an indication for its performance' (Sir William Heneage Ogilvie, British surgeon).

Marshall BJ, Warren JR (June 1984). "Unidentified curved bacilli in the stomach of patients with gastritis and peptic ulceration".

The Lancet. 323 (8390):1311-5.
Biopsy specimens were taken from intact areas of antral mucosa in 100 consecutive consenting patients presenting for gastroscopy. Spiral or curved bacilli were demonstrated in specimens from 58 patients. Bacilli cultured from 11 of these biopsies were gram-negative, flagellate, and microaerophilic and appeared to be a new species related to the genus Campylobacter. The bacteria were present in almost all patients with active chronic gastritis, duodenal ulcer, or gastric ulcer and thus may be an important factor in the aetiology of these diseases.

Upper Gastro intestinal Bleeding

This used to be a common general surgical emergency; however, the progress of endoscopic interventions has now made surgical interventions less frequent.

The presentation can be acute with sudden onset of melaena or haematemesis. Melaena is the passage of stools that are schwarz (black; German), smelly, slimy, and sticky (the four S's) due to breakdown of haemoglobin to acid haematin by the products of digestion. The principles of management are directed towards stabilisation of the patient. This is then followed by localisation of the causative pathology followed by medical management for most patients. When that fails, the next step is endoscopic management. Surgical management is reserved for the few that fail endoscopic management.

Gastro-oesophageal bleeding can be related to aspirin and non-steroidal use in about a third of the patients. The bleeding is due to weakening of the mucosal barrier brought about by inhibition of cyclo-oxygenase and consequent decrease in the production of prostacyclin. Prostacyclin protects the mucosa by increasing mucous and bicarbonate secretion.

The other major causes include the following:

- Gastro-oesophageal varices
- Stress ulcerations
- Longitudinal Mallory Weiss tear of the Oesophago-gastric junction due to retching and vomiting

Endoscopic Therapy for Peptic Ulcer Bleeding

- Adrenaline injection to slow bleeding but not very effective in isolation
- Thermal modalities—heater probes, bipolar coagulation
- Clips—more recently over the scope clips
- Hemospray

Treatment of Oesophageal Varices

- Band ligation of varices
- Propranolol or other non-selective beta blockers
- Thrombin injections for gastric varices
- Somatostatin/Terilipressin
- Balloon Tamponade
- Trans-jugular intra hepatic porta-systemic shunts (TIPSS)

ACUTE APPENDICITIS

Acute appendicitis is a common abdominal emergency.

The presentation is normally with nausea and vomiting. These are a reflex to autonomic pain and generally follow onset of pain; most people have no desire to eat. A low-grade pyrexia and an elevated white cell count and CRP are but manifestations of systemic inflammation and the body's response to it.

Common presenting symptoms of acute appendicitis are as follows:

- Central abdominal pain
- Nausea (reflex to pain)
- Vomiting (just once or twice)
- Pyrexia
- Localised pain in right lower quadrant

Migrating Pain

Classically, the pain in appendicitis appears to migrate from being central at onset, to the right iliac fossa when the disease is more established. This is because the appendix is part of the mid gut, and this autonomic pain is poorly localised and felt in the umbilical region. As inflammation progresses, it involves the abdominal muscles and irritates the somatic nerves. Somatic pain is more direct and localised. As the appendix lies deep to the abdominal muscles in the right iliac fossa the inflammation of the parietal layer of the peritoneum involves the abdominal muscles that are innervated by somatic nerves and presents as localised pain. The worsening pain is then located overlying the appendix and thus in the right iliac fossa.

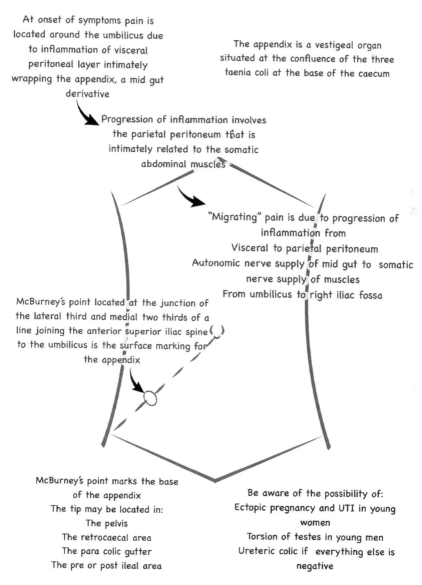

At onset of symptoms pain is located around the umbilicus due to inflammation of visceral peritoneal layer intimately wrapping the appendix, a mid gut derivative

The appendix is a vestigeal organ situated at the confluence of the three taenia coli at the base of the caecum

Progression of inflammation involves the parietal peritoneum that is intimately related to the somatic abdominal muscles

"Migrating" pain is due to progression of inflammation from
Visceral to parietal peritoneum
Autonomic nerve supply of mid gut to somatic nerve supply of muscles
From umbilicus to right iliac fossa

McBurney's point located at the junction of the lateral third and medial two thirds of a line joining the anterior superior iliac spine ( ) to the umbilicus is the surface marking for the appendix

McBurney's point marks the base of the appendix
The tip may be located in:
The pelvis
The retrocaecal area
The para colic gutter
The pre or post ileal area

Be aware of the possibility of:
Ectopic pregnancy and UTI in young women
Torsion of testes in young men
Ureteric colic if everything else is negative

Figure 7: Key features of appendicular inflammation

Pain that is felt at the outset is due to the irritation of the visceral layer of the peritoneum that is closely applied to the viscera, much like a cling film wrapper. The nerve supply for this is predominantly autonomic. Pain that is felt subsequently and sequentially is due to irritation of the somatic layer of the peritoneum that is adjacent to the musculature of the abdomen. The irritation of the muscle layer leads to guarding and to rebound tenderness. It is localised in the right iliac fossa.

Differences between autonomic and somatic types of pain

Viscera is of endodermal origin and has an autonomic innervation. It manifests as 'Autonomic pain'	The pain is diffuse and thus difficult to localise; it manifests as gripes and cramps	Distension and stretch, but not cut or incision causes pain; stretch of flatulence but not cut of polypectomy causes pain
Ectodermal structures such as musculature, bone and skin are innervated by somatic nerves. It manifests as 'somatic pain'	This pain is localised; sharp and can be severe	Fractures of bones, injury and incision to skin and muscles can cause localised pain

Embryological parts of the gut

Fore Gut	Mid-Gut	Hind Gut
Extends from the mouth to the ampulla of Vater	Extends from the ampulla of Vater to proximal two-thirds of transverse colon	Extends from the distal third of transverse colon to rectum
This includes the stomach, proximal duodenum, liver, spleen	This includes, the ileum, jejunum, appendix, caecum, ascending colon, and the proximal two-thirds of transverse colon	This includes the distal third of the transverse colon, descending colon, sigmoid colon, and rectum
Coeliac artery supplies the fore gut	Superior mesenteric artery supplies the mid gut	Inferior mesenteric artery supplies the hind gut
Pain can be manifest across the epigastrium	Pain tends to be in the umbilical region	Pain presents in the hypogastrium or supra pubic area

Appendicular Mass

The mass that accompanies appendicular inflammation normally presents itself in about forty-eight hours after the onset of symptoms. This occurs because the body's response to inflammation tries to isolate and contain the spread of inflammation to the rest of the abdominal cavity. The pathophysiology of this process primarily involves the greater omentum which serves to protect the spread of inflammation.

This localisation occurs when the omentum [abdominal policeman] and adjacent loops of bowel combine forces and wall off the 'troublemaker'. This process is common to all types of pathology that need containment such as cholecystitis, diverticulitis, appendicitis, visceral perforation, and salpingitis. The inflamed organ that is enveloped by the omentum, bowel, as well as any adjacent organ like the uterus or even the ovary manifests as a tender mass.

If a faecolith obstructs the lumen of the appendix, a closed loop obstruction occurs. The secretions of the mucosa of the appendix being obstructed causes the appendix to distend. This can lead to perforation rapidly (within twelve to twenty-four hours) causing localised or generalised peritonitis.

When localisation fails, there is generalisation of the peritoneal irritation leading to peritonitis. This process may fail in the very young and the very old. In the very young due to under development of omentum and in the elderly due to its atrophy.

The progressive inflammation can lead to formation of an abscess. This presents as increasing pain and fluctuating fever that is referred to as the 'thicket fence' fever due to the up and down course of the body temperature. It must be noted that a similar effect is produced with paracetamol as its effect can intermittently decrease the body temperature even in patients with a steady temperature.

In young women, pain in the right lower quadrant of the abdomen may be due to pelvic inflammatory disease, retrograde menstruation or mid cycle ovulation pain referred to as Mittleschmerz.

Appendicitis End Response

- Resolution
- Mass formation—localisation
- Abscess formation
- Peritonitis
- Fibrosis

In all young women presenting with abdominal pain a menstrual history as well as the contraceptive status with measurement of Beta HCG is mandatory. A history of oral contraceptive use must always be obtained.

The urine must be examined for nitrates which when positive, will favour a urinary infection.

Conservative management of localised peritonitis in young women may affect tubal patency increasing the risk of ectopic pregnancy subsequently. It is therefore important to consider early intervention or laparoscopy in young women with suspected pelvic inflammation.

If appendicular abscess, perforation, or gangrene is noted at operation, then forty-eight hours or more of antibiotics is indicated. A common organism that is present in appendicular inflammation is Bacteroides, and this is treated with metronidazole; the other common organisms are E. coli and Klebsiella, and antibiotic treatment will be needed as per your hospital protocol.

Inflammatory bowel disease such as Crohn's must also be borne in mind when the history and presentation are not very clear, and the patient offers a history of diarrhoea.

A diagnosis is not always possible, and 'nonspecific abdominal pain' is acceptable as a discharge diagnosis and leaves open the possibility of considering other diagnosis at a later date if the problem recurs.

In the elderly patients presenting with acute right iliac pain and a palpable mass, a CT scan will be needed to exclude caecal or even appendicular malignancies.

> If the appendix is normal at operation and no abnormalities are noted in the bowel, pelvic organs including the ovaries and if Meckel's is excluded, then renal and ureteric pathology such as calculi must be ruled out prior to discharge with further imaging.

Imaging as an aid to diagnosis in Appendicitis

- Ultrasound scan is non invasive but it requires a radiologist with appropriate skills to make a diagnosis of appendicitis. It can be favoured in the younger patients as it avoids radiation.
- CT scan of the abdomen has a 96% specificity and the advantage of ruling out other pelvic causes for the presentation. This is favoured in the elderly and the obese.
- MRI of the abdomen is a useful tool in select patients where a clear diagnosis needs confirmation.

Surgical Management

The principles of general management as laid out previously must be implemented prior to a decision to operate.

Appendicectomies are mostly done laparoscopically rather than with open surgery. Laparoscopic surgery facilitates early discharge as there is reduced pain and discomfort compared to an open operation. The open operation may be needed in the presence of a mass or when converting to an open operation following failed laparoscopic attempt. Traditionally, the incision for open appendicectomy overlies the **McBurney** point. The exposure is through a **'grid iron'** incision that splits the muscle fibres of the abdominal wall along the long axis of the muscles instead of cutting across them. When the exposure with the 'grid iron' incision is insufficient, then the muscles of the abdominal wall are divided in a process referred to as the **'Rutherford Morrison'** extension after the surgeon who popularised it.

Complications such as **appendicular abscesses** can be drained radiologically prior to an interval appendicectomy later.

In the presence of an **appendicular mass**, a non-operative management with resolution of the mass will permit an interval appendicectomy.

Where an immediate appendicectomy is not carried out or deferred for reasons of complications then an **interval appendicectomy** may need consideration in 6-12 weeks after resolution. A MRI scan of the abdomen will reveal the location and presence of the appendicitis prior to such intervention. In a small number of patients, the original inflammation and the process of fibrosis may destroy the appendix rendering the interval appendicectomy superfluous.

It is mandatory to **check the histology** and ensure confirmation of appendicitis. Rarely, you might come across a diagnosis of carcinoma, carcinoid, or Crohn's of the appendix. Those patients will need discussion regarding further management.

Differential Diagnosis

- Pelvic inflammatory disease
- Meckel's diverticulitis
- Crohn's disease
- Carcinoid of the appendix
- Adeno carcinoma of the caecum/appendix
- Ureteric calculi
- Diverticulitis of the sigmoid
- Ectopic pregnancy
- Torsion of the testis
- Amoebic typhlitis or amoeboma
- Ileo-caecal tuberculosis

Case-Based Discussion

Because appendicitis is a common surgical problem, it is important to have a clear understanding of the management. It is useful to work out a plan of management for the following possible presentations:

- Right iliac pain in a ten-year-old girl
  - Clinical assessment
  - Routine bloods
  - Imaging with ultrasound /CT scan

- Appendicectomy on confirmation of diagnosis
- Non operative management with re assessment and review when appendicitis is not confirmed
- Lower abdominal pain in a thirty-year-old lady
  - Additional to the above
  - urinary nitrates and microscopy
  - Possible laparoscopic exploration if imaging is not confirmatory
  - Involvement of the gynaecological team to exclude PID
- Presentation after forty-eight hours of onset of symptoms when there is a palpable mass in the right iliac fossa
  - Define the presence or absence of a mass in the right lower quadrant of the abdomen
  - Exclude malignancy where appropriate
  - Surgical or conservative management depending on the level of expertise available and the fitness of the patient
  - Conservative management will include active monitoring of system and mass. Treatment with antibiotics and intravenous fluids. Switching to surgery if the mass fails to resolve.
- Presentation with generalised abdominal tenderness and rigidity
  - A CT scan will be needed to exclude peritonitis.
  - Laparotomy rather than exploration with cosmetic incisions is preferred
  - Critical care team must be involved in the post-operative care as the sepsis may have a delayed manifestation of over 6 to 12 hours post-surgical intervention
  - Needless to say cultures must be obtained at surgery and appropriate antibiotic therapy instituted
- Right iliac pain with microscopic haematuria
  - Urinary infection and ureteric calculi must be excluded
- Presence of fever and sore throat prior to presentation with pain tends to occur in children. In these cases, the paediatric team must be involved in the decision making as the presentation may not be that of an acute appendicitis.

HERNIA

Abdominal wall hernia
1. Epigastric
2. Umbilical/para umbilical
3. Spigelian
4. Incisional
5. Inguinal
6. Femoral
7. Lumbar

Hernia is defined as protrusion of viscus or part of a viscus from the cavity which contains it to the exterior or to another cavity

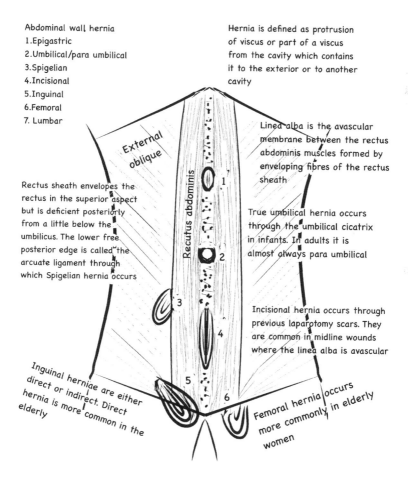

Rectus sheath envelopes the rectus in the superior aspect but is deficient posteriorly from a little below the umbilicus. The lower free posterior edge is called the arcuate ligament through which Spigelian hernia occurs

Linea alba is the avascular membrane between the rectus abdominis muscles formed by enveloping fibres of the rectus sheath

True umbilical hernia occurs through the umbilical cicatrix in infants. In adults it is almost always para umbilical

Incisional hernia occurs through previous laparotomy scars. They are common in midline wounds where the linea alba is avascular

Inguinal herniae are either direct or indirect. Direct hernia is more common in the elderly

Femoral hernia occurs more commonly in elderly women

Rectus muscle can move apart with increasing abdominal girth, stretching and weakening the linea alba. This is called divarication. On sitting up the linea bulges but there is no defect in the membrane, only a weakness

Figure 8: Various types of hernia

A hernia is protrusion of viscus or part of a viscus from the cavity in which it is contained to another cavity or to the exterior. It stands to reason that they can occur wherever there is a body cavity including the cranium, thorax, and abdomen.

Umbilical Hernia

An umbilical hernia is generally congenital and occurs through the true umbilical cicatrix. They are common in children and seldom need intervention till the age of three years by which time a sizable portion would have resolved without need for surgical intervention.

In adults the defect in the umbilical region is outside the true umbilicus and is referred to as para-umbilical hernia. They are symptomless in many patients.

Para-umbilical Hernia—predisposing factors

- Pregnancy
- Abdominal exercise
- Cirrhosis
- Ascites

Incisional Hernia

These arise in scars of incisions for abdominal operations and are therefore called Incisional hernia. They can occur anywhere in the abdomen where there is a scar. They are more common when there is a history of a previous wound infection but are also noted in the obese and the emaciated where there are problems with healing.

Predisposing factors for incisional hernia include the following:

- High BMI
- Low BMI

- Diabetic
- COPD
- Previously Infected wounds
- Nutritionally compromised

Divarication of the Rectus Abdominis Muscle

Divarication is not a hernia. Divarication occurs due to the recti muscles moving apart either due to multiple pregnancies, obesity, or both. The linea alba, an avascular membranous layer in between the two rectus muscles, stretches apart as the rectus moves apart with abdominal distendion. It then becomes weak over time and can present as a bulge. This bulge becomes obvious when the patient changes posture from lying to sitting up but disappears when the patient stands unlike a hernia. A hernial bulge will become prominent when the patient stands up, but a divarication does not. In a hernia, there is a defect, and contents protrude through the defect. In a divarication, there is no defect, and there is no risk of strangulation. It does not require surgery unless for cosmetic reasons.

Inguinal Hernia

Inguinal hernia occurs in the inguinal canal. It can be either a direct or an indirect hernia. The inguinal canal is a potential space that extends almost transversely from the internal ring to the external ring.

The boundaries are as follows:

Anteriorly: External oblique laterally and the conjoint fibres of internal and transverse abdominis in the medial part
Posteriorly: The transversalis fascia
Inferiorly: The inguinal ligament
Superiorly: The arching fibres of the conjoint tendon

It is worth bearing in mind that evolution appears not to have caught up with the new anatomy when the human beings became bipedal from being quadrupedal. This means the thigh, which supports the lower abdomen in a quadruped, has moved away from the lower abdomen in a biped as the straightening of the torso evolved. This single change has left an unsupported space, in the lower abdomen below the arcuate line that has been filled in by loose areolar tissue and transversalis fascia instead of a muscular structure such as the posterior rectus sheath. Thus, there is an area of weakness through which a direct hernia can occur.

Commonly, the direct hernia occurs due to muscle failure, and consequently the patient is likely to be elderly. It seldom descends into the scrotum, although the bulge may overlie the proximal scrotum purely because of the effect of size.

Indirect hernia, by contrast, traverses the internal ring and protrudes along the inguinal canal and through the external ring into the scrotum when it is large. Any hernia that is in the scrotum enveloping the testis is an indirect hernia. It has a significant degree of a congenital element to it and hence is more common in younger people.

Predisposing Factors

Factors that cause a sudden increase in intra-abdominal pressure can lead to hernia. In the young and fit persons playing football, rugby, or tennis where one twists and turns actively during the game, a sudden increase in pressure can lead to tears in the muscles around the groin.

Jerry Gilmore, who initially drew attention to the link between sports injury and hernia, stated that the pathology of Gilmore's Groin is as follows:

- Torn external oblique aponeurosis
- Torn conjoined tendon
- Conjoined tendon torn from pubic tubercle
- Dehiscence between conjoined tendon and inguinal ligament

Apart from this, the other factors include the following:

- Chronic cough—secondary to COPD or bronchiectasis
- Chronic constipation
- Prostatism with straining at micturition
- Increase in intra-abdominal pressure due to muscular activity, ascites, and more, leading to umbilical, incisional, and inguinal hernia

A good history from the patient must therefore include a discussion about the possible predisposing causes and attempts must be made to alleviate constipation or cough prior to surgery; in some cases, prostatic surgery may be needed before considering a repair of the hernia.

The anterior superior iliac spine is the first bony prominence encountered as the hand is slid laterally along the Inguinal ligament. It is the lateral attachment of the Inguinal ligament

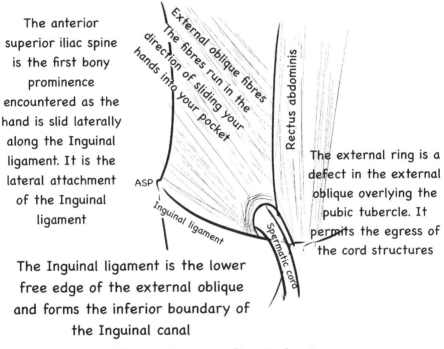

External oblique fibres
The fibres run in the direction of sliding your hands into your pocket

Rectus abdominis

ASP

Inguinal ligament

Spermatic cord

The external ring is a defect in the external oblique overlying the pubic tubercle. It permits the egress of the cord structures

The Inguinal ligament is the lower free edge of the external oblique and forms the inferior boundary of the Inguinal canal

Figure 9: Anatomy of inguinal region

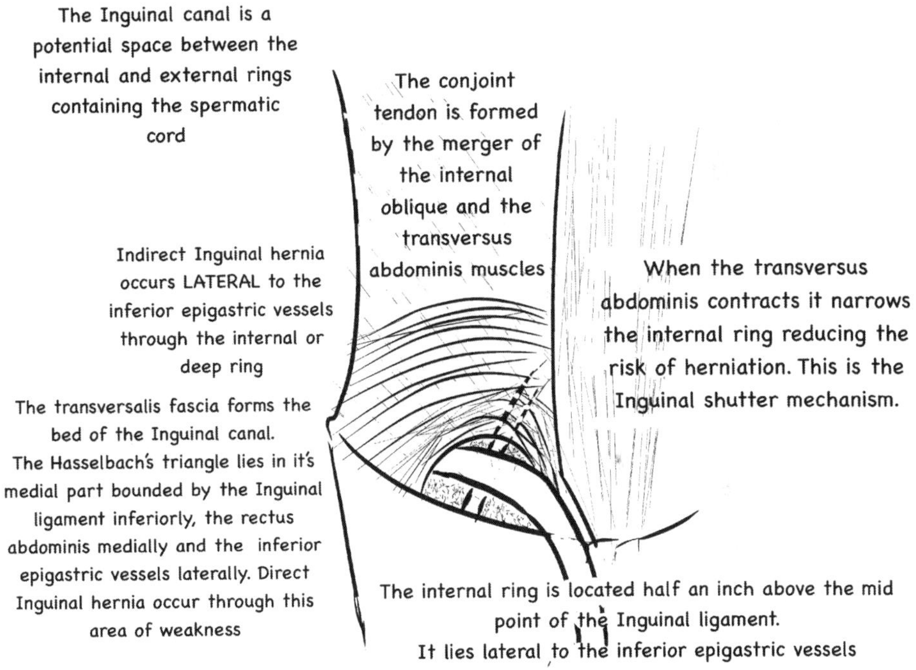

The Inguinal canal is a potential space between the internal and external rings containing the spermatic cord

The conjoint tendon is formed by the merger of the internal oblique and the transversus abdominis muscles

Indirect Inguinal hernia occurs LATERAL to the inferior epigastric vessels through the internal or deep ring

When the transversus abdominis contracts it narrows the internal ring reducing the risk of herniation. This is the Inguinal shutter mechanism.

The transversalis fascia forms the bed of the Inguinal canal. The Hasselbach's triangle lies in it's medial part bounded by the Inguinal ligament inferiorly, the rectus abdominis medially and the inferior epigastric vessels laterally. Direct Inguinal hernia occur through this area of weakness

The internal ring is located half an inch above the mid point of the Inguinal ligament. It lies lateral to the inferior epigastric vessels

Figure 10: Inguinal shutter mechanism and anatomy

Examination

When a patient presents with a lump in the groin, it is important to define if it is an inguinal or a femoral hernia. The neck of the inguinal hernia will be above and lateral to the pubic tubercle. The neck of the femoral hernia will be below and lateral to the pubic tubercle. The exception is when a femoral hernia becomes large, it flops back on itself like a lazy U due to the fascial attachments across the femoral triangle. It can then lie across the inguinal ligament instead of following gravity. The fascial attachments prevent the hernia from descending to the knee

If it is an inguinal hernia, then it is important to clarify whether it is of the direct or the indirect type. Herniae that occur through the Hesselbach's triangle is referred to as a direct hernia. When it protrudes through the internal ring and takes an oblique route, is referred to as indirect in type. Because of the obliquity and as it protrudes through the internal ring where it can be constricted (neck of sac), there is a greater risk of strangulation. Advice therefore favours surgery than observation.

If the bulge is not clinically obvious at the outset, then it is best to make the patient stand up for initial inspection. Asking the patient to stand up and cough will generally make the bulge obvious.

Classically, to define the type of inguinal hernia, the hernia should be reduced with the patient lying down. The internal ring can then be compressed with one hand, and the patient is asked to stand up and cough whilst the internal ring remains compressed by the hand. If the coughing causes the hernia to protrude despite adequate compression of the internal ring, then obviously it is not protruding through the internal ring, and thus it is a direct rather than an indirect hernia.

The hernia repairs being similar for both indirect and direct types it is right to ask why one should ever need to make this distinction. This distinction is necessary as the advice given may vary according to the fitness of the patient for surgical intervention. Risk of strangulation is higher in an indirect hernia. Advice on indirect hernia therefore may well be early surgery rather that the wait and watch policy that may be undertaken for the elderly patients with a direct hernia and multiple comorbidities. Almost all herniae grow larger with time.

The reason for surgery is either for the prevention of progression and occurrence of complications or for complications.

Increasingly, commonly we see patients with a reducible hernia but with pain. That too may be a relative indication for surgical intervention. Whilst by and large a hernia is a clinical diagnosis, there are circumstances when investigations are needed.

Complications of Inguinal Hernia

- **Pain**—multifactorial but could be due to muscle tear in early hernia to possible narrowing at the neck or compression
- **Irreducibility**—due to adhesions between contents and the sac or intrasaccular adhesions of contents making it globular and thus difficult to reduce. Forcible reduction of these 'reduction en masse' along with the sac may cause strangulation later if the sac constricts the contents
- **Obstruction**—rarely a feature without irreducibility or strangulation
- **Strangulation**—more common with indirect hernia when the neck constricts around a sac containing loops of bowel. Initially it compromises venous supply leading to swelling and raised intra saccular pressure and then to arterial compromise causing gangrene of the bowel

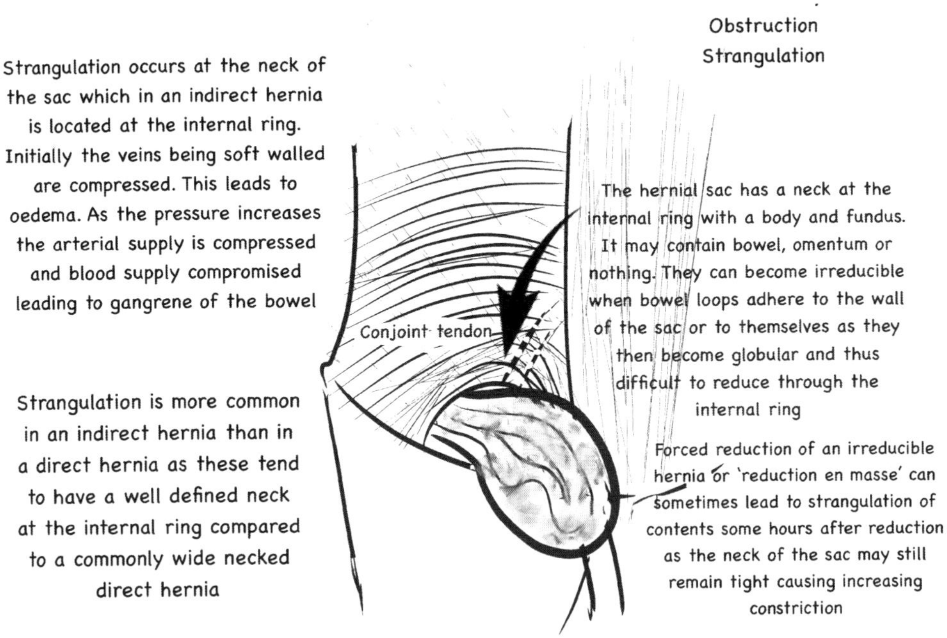

Strangulation occurs at the neck of the sac which in an indirect hernia is located at the internal ring. Initially the veins being soft walled are compressed. This leads to oedema. As the pressure increases the arterial supply is compressed and blood supply compromised leading to gangrene of the bowel

Strangulation is more common in an indirect hernia than in a direct hernia as these tend to have a well defined neck at the internal ring compared to a commonly wide necked direct hernia

Obstruction
Strangulation

The hernial sac has a neck at the internal ring with a body and fundus. It may contain bowel, omentum or nothing. They can become irreducible when bowel loops adhere to the wall of the sac or to themselves as they then become globular and thus difficult to reduce through the internal ring

Forced reduction of an irreducible hernia or 'reduction en masse' can sometimes lead to strangulation of contents some hours after reduction as the neck of the sac may still remain tight causing increasing constriction

Conjoint tendon

Figure 11: The hernial sac

Investigations

A dynamic ultrasound scan may be needed when the presence of a hernia is not definable clinically, but the patient offers a good history for a hernia. The sonographer will then be able to demonstrate the presence of a hernia by asking the patient to cough or perform the Valsalva manoeuvre during the time of scanning.

A recent meta-analysis of USS ('sonography') in the diagnosis of inguinal hernias found 9 articles that matched their inclusion criteria. Pooled data showed a sensitivity of ultrasound of 87.3%, a specificity of 85.5%, and a positive predictive value of 73.6% i.e., a patient with a positive ultrasound report has a 73.6% chance of having an inguinal hernia

Robinson, A., et al., A systematic review and meta-analysis of the role of radiology in the diagnosis of occult inguinal hernia. Surg Endosc, 2013. 27(1): p. 11-8

Magnetic resonance imaging (MRI) may be needed if the patient has groin pain without an obvious hernia. This is done not only to outline the presence or absence of a hernia but also to exclude muscular tears or hip-related problems.

A CT scan of the abdomen is also another option, but on occasions if the hernia is fully reduced, it may not be picked up on the scan in the supine position. This is true in theory rather than in practice. CT also distinguishes between an inguinal and femoral hernia. Obviously when there is obstruction, a CT is carried out prior to laparotomy more often to exclude other pathologies in the abdomen and to define the level and seriousness of the pathology pertaining to the obstruction.

Management

It is important to discuss with all patients the following:

- Surgery versus no surgery—that is, wait and watch as opposed to operative surgery
- Laparoscopic versus open surgery
- Loco-regional versus general anaesthesia for surgery

The recommendation of the hernia society is to consider surgical intervention in asymptomatic patients under sixty-five years of age and in symptomatic patients over sixty-five years of age.

Laparoscopic surgery is preferred for bilateral hernia and for recurrence after previous open or laparoscopic surgery.

For unilateral hernia, it is a matter for discussion with the patient as to the various options.

In the elderly with comorbidities, repair under local anaesthesia or regional anaesthesia is preferable.

Children under the age of sixteen years should be treated by the paediatric surgeons.

Hernia in infants should be treated urgently. The prior rule used to be 'never send a new born baby home with a hernia unless a herniotomy is carried out'.

Operations for Inguinal Hernia

Operations for inguinal hernia have now been simplified with the introduction of tension-free mesh repair. In the past, the inguinal canal used to be obliterated by approximating the 'roof to the floor'. The conjoint tendon used to be approximated to the inguinal ligament under tension! Post-operative pain was the norm, and patients used to stay in hospital for up to a week. The most popular operation was the Bassini repair with a recurrence rate of 12 per cent or more. With the advent of tension-free mesh repairs either laparoscopically or open, the defect is bridged over by the mesh without any forceful approximation. As in normal life, so in operations; the absence of tension augers well!

Notoras was one of the first persons to draw attention to the mesh repair for inguinal hernia.

Experience with Mersilene Mesh in Abdominal Wall Repair by M J Notaras FRCS (Department of Surgery, University College Hospital, London and Barnet General Hospital, London)
MJ Notaras - 1974 - journals.sagepub.com

The operation carried out with mesh goes by the name of Lichtenstein after he published his results of a massive number of hernia repairs.

The American Journal of Surgery

Volume 153, Issue 6, June 1987, Pages 553-559
Herniorrhaphy: A personal experience with 6,321 cases
Irving L. Lichtenstein MD, FACS1

Abstract
The results of 6,321 consecutive herniorrhaphies have been reported. Over 20 percent of the cases were referred recurrences when first seen. Ninety-one percent of the patients were followed from 2 to 14 years, with an overall recurrence rate of 0.7 percent. A low recurrence rate was not unfavourably affected by the prompt resumption of activity post-operatively. Some recurrences are unavoidable; however, it is essential to accept the dictum that all hernias can be cured.

Femoral Hernia

This is more common in women than men. This hernia is also one that is commonly missed in routine clinical examinations, especially in the presence of central obesity. 'No examination of the abdomen is complete without examination of the hernial sites.' This adage becomes obvious in any acute presentation of intestinal obstruction in the absence of an obvious cause such as previous operations. In patients with a high BMI, the groin fold is difficult to define, and the hernia can be missed easily leading to strangulation later. It is also not surprising that often the elderly patient may have failed to notice it themselves. This hernia, in the elderly, has a high risk of mortality of up to 30 per cent when it strangulates; timely detection and action, as always, will reduce the morbidity and mortality.

Location and Anatomy

Femoral herniae are located below and lateral to the pubic tubercle. The following are boundaries of the hernia:

- Anteriorly: The inguinal ligament
- Posteriorly: The pectinate ligament
- Medially: The lacunar ligament
- Laterally: The femoral vein

The hernia is located in the femoral canal that forms part of the femoral sheath as outlined in figure 12. The femoral sheath is the fascial layer that invests the femoral vessels as they leave the abdomen and proceed to the limb.

Like all herniae, the complications of a femoral hernia include obstruction and strangulation. In most cases, the content is only fatty tissue, however when there is bowel in it, the risk of strangulation becomes greater. A very small proportion of femoral hernia are completely reducible. The risk of obstruction and strangulation is high, so surgery is normally recommended in the fit patient.

Femoral hernia occurs more commonly in elderly women.

Indirect hernia and femoral hernia have a higher risk of strangulation.

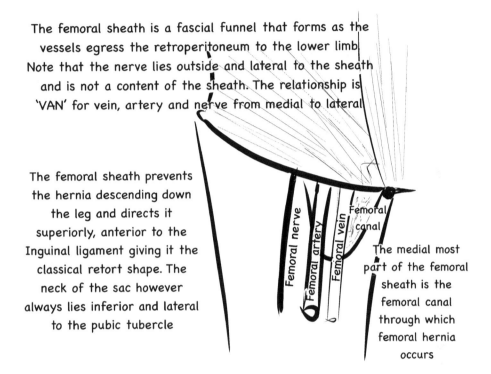

The femoral sheath is a fascial funnel that forms as the vessels egress the retroperitoneum to the lower limb. Note that the nerve lies outside and lateral to the sheath and is not a content of the sheath. The relationship is 'VAN' for vein, artery and nerve from medial to lateral

The femoral sheath prevents the hernia descending down the leg and directs it superiorly, anterior to the Inguinal ligament giving it the classical retort shape. The neck of the sac however always lies inferior and lateral to the pubic tubercle

Femoral nerve

Femoral artery

Femoral vein

Femoral canal

The medial most part of the femoral sheath is the femoral canal through which femoral hernia occurs

Figure 12: Femoral hernia

Repair of Femoral Hernia after Excision of Sac

- Low repair of Lockwood—Accessing from below the inguinal ligament and approximating the anterior wall (Inguinal ligament) to the posterior wall (pectinate or Cooper's ligament). 'Roof to floor' repair.
- High repair of Lotheissen—The approach is from above the inguinal ligament in the pre-peritoneal plane.
- AK Henry—Repair is carried out with a vertical incision over inguinal region. This is now defunct.
- Laparotomy or Laparoscopic repair.

Mesh repair is increasingly more common, although in the elderly, a low repair of Lockwood is possible with or without a mesh.

In all these repairs, it must be borne in mind that the femoral vein lies in close proximity to the neck of the sac. The vein must not only be protected from injury but also from being narrowed. Narrowing the vein can lead to problems with venous drainage of the leg.

Emergency Operations

These can be technically difficult because the bowel may be distended, ischaemic, and prone to tear on traction. Repairs from above the inguinal ligament through a laparotomy or pre-peritoneal plane is preferred, with mobilisation being carried out after proximal and distal clamping of bowel prior to traction. Many of the patients presenting with strangulated femoral hernia are elderly with comorbidities. The mortality from a strangulated femoral hernia in elderly women can be very high. The post-operative care will need management in a level two setting for most.

VARICOSE VEINS

Varicose veins are:
Elongated
Tortuous
Thin walled veins

Varicose veins commonly affect the long and short saphenous veins of the lower limb

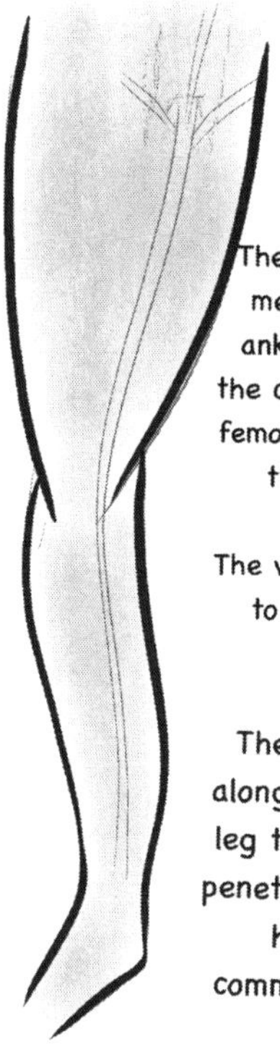

There are perforating veins that direct the flow from the superficial to the deep veins that run along the femoral and tibial arteries
There are three of them in the medial aspect of the leg located a hand's breadth above the medial malleolus, a hand's breadth below and above the knee

The long saphenous vein runs along the medial aspect of the lower limb from ankle to groin where it passes through the cribriform fascia to enter the common femoral vein. Three named tributaries join the vein prior to it penetrating the cribriform fascia.
The vein has a number of valves that seek to direct the flow towards the heart

The short saphenous vein runs along the posterior aspect of the leg to enter the popliteal vein by penetrating the popliteal fascia. It has perforator veins that communicate with the deep veins

TED or thromboembolic deterrent stockings are graduated compression stockings that compress the superficial veins of the lower limbs thus directing the blood to the deep veins. This increases the flow thorough the deep veins. This simple measure decreases the risk of DVT in the post operative period

Figure 13: Anatomy of the long saphenous vein

Pathophysiology

Varicosities occur in a vein due to the thinning of the wall. This leads to dilatation, and as the valves remain the same size, they appear to move apart, causing them to dysfunction and permit retrograde flow.

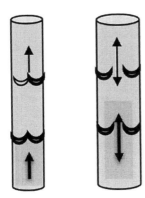

The increase in the diameter of the vein increases the circumference and thus moves the valves apart causing retrograde flow

Retrograde flow in the veins raises the back pressure on the venous side of the capillaries. The Starling pressures at the capillary level are altered because of this venous hypertension.

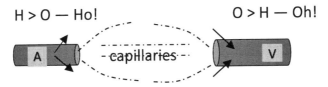

H = hydrostatic pressure; O = osmotic pressure;
A = arteriolar end; V = venular end

Hydrostatic pressure is higher than osmotic pressure at the arteriolar end of the capillaries; hence, the net flow is outwards at the arteriolar end.

Osmotic pressure is higher than hydrostatic pressure at the venular end of the capillaries; hence, the net flow is inwards at the venular end.

Venous obstruction due one factor or another can alter this basic equation. When it does, the inflow at the venous end becomes less than the outflow into the capillaries at the arterial end. This reduction of inflow at the venular end, causes stagnation in the capillary region. This will cause oedema.

Pathophysiology of Venous Hypertension

There are approximately eighteen valves in the long saphenous vein. These valves meet in the midline and effectively permit flow in one direction, always towards the heart.

Due to possibly an inherited weakness in the weave of the wall of the vein, the veins start to dilate over time. This can also occur due to obstruction to flow leading to stretching of the wall of the vein. When the diameter of the vein starts to increase, the valves move away from each other. When this happens, the direction of flow is reversed and the valves start to leak. Once the leakage starts, it is progressive and causes more and more distension distally. As there are no valves in the main veins of the body such as the IVC, the backwards pressure at the venous end increases and will be equal to the height of the column of blood in the vein from the heart to the foot. This can be as much as a 100 mmHg.

This is venous hypertension. Venous hypertension reduces influx of fluid at the venular end of the capillaries as the hydrostatic pressure now exceeds the osmotic pressure.

Capillary leakage occurs at the arterial end and causes RBCs to efflux into the interstitial tissue. The RBCs may not all be able to re-enter at the venular end and are left behind in the peri capillary tissue. The RBCs are broken down by macrophages, and hemosiderin is deposited around the arterioles, causing 'peri vascular cuffing' leading to pigmentation and lipodermatosclerosis.

This pathological process impedes delivery of oxygen, which in turn leads to breakdown of tissue, causing ulceration. When the ulcers heal, they cause fibrosis. Fibrosis around the ankle restricts movement, and reduced movement at the ankle reduces calf muscle movement and failure of the Soleal muscle pump, a force that assists blood flow back to the heart. A vicious cycle then sets in, with more peripheral pooling, more pigmentation, and further ulceration. All are consequences of varicose veins that result in venous hypertension.

Progressive Effects of Venous Hypertension

- Greater efflux at the arteriolar end
- RBCs leak into the pericapillary space
- RBCs are broken down by macrophages to haemosiderin
- Haemosiderin is deposited around capillaries
- Pigmentation and perivascular cuffing occur
- This leads to decreased oxygen delivery to tissues
- Results in breakdown of skin and ulceration around ankle
- Attempt at healing leads to fibrosis around ankle
- Restricts ankle movements
- Leads to failure of Soleal muscle pump
- Vicious cycle sets in

Complications of Venous Hypertension

- Leg ulcers
- Lipodermatosclerosis
- Pigmentation
- Bleeding
- Ankle stiffness

Thin vessels that are dilated can bleed spontaneously because of the venous hypertension or after minor trauma. If they do the best, immediate treatment is elevation and compression.

The leg ulcers are very difficult to treat and seldom heal despite the best efforts of compression and elevation. They occur close to the ankle because of the location of the long saphenous vein. Stiffness of the ankle reduces the efficiency of the calf muscle pump. The venous stagnation worsens as the 'vis a tergo', or push from behind towards the heart, fails. This sets up a perpetually worsening cycle. Mobility of the ankle is the key to success in all venous problems affecting the legs but can seldom be achieved.

Assessment and Treatment

Historically, the varicose veins of the legs were assessed by looking for incompetence at the Sapheno femoral (long saphenous) or Saphenopopliteal (short saphenous) junctions. There can also be incompetence of perforators. Three such perforators are located along the long saphenous vein.

- A hand's breadth above the ankle
- A hand's breadth below the knee
- A hand's breadth above the knee

Normal Direction of Flow in the Saphenous Veins

- In the long and short saphenous veins, the normal direction of flow is always from the ankle towards the heart, that is, from distal to proximal
- In the perforators the normal flow is always from superficial to deep

Direction of Flow in Varicose Saphenous Veins

- With onset of venous hypertension secondary to incompetence of the valves, there is a reversal of the flow.
- This leads to retrograde flow from the heart to the legs in the main saphenous veins
- From deep to superficial in the perforating veins

Traditionally, in the days before Doppler, Trendelenburg recommended identifying the retrograde flow at the Sapheno-femoral junction by the following steps.

- Lie the patient down
- Elevate the limb
- Empty the veins of blood
- Compress the saphenofemoral junction
- Stand the patient up with continued compression

- Release the compression in the upright posture
- Observe the filling of the vein
- Immediate retrograde filling denotes a positive test

Doppler has made this defunct, and we now check for 'to and fro' sounds with a Doppler probe at the sapheno-femoral junction by squeezing (prograde flow) and releasing the compression of the calf muscles (retrograde flow). Normally on compression of the calf, there is a prograde flow with a recorded Doppler sound. On release of compression, if the valve is competent, there is no retrograde flow and thus no recorded sound. When the valve is incompetent there is a whoosh sound on compression and whoosh sound on release—a *whoosh-whoosh* instead of just one *whoosh*!

Perforator incompetence is likewise determined by demonstrating the flow pattern. When they are incompetent, the direction of flow is reversed, and the flow is from the deep to the superficial veins.

Trendelenburg Operation–Long Saphenous Varicosity

The dictat used to be, 'Trendelenburg test positive—Trendelenburg operation. Trendelenburg test negative—no Trendelenburg operation.'

Typically, for the long saphenous varicosity, the operation entails ligation of the long saphenous vein at the sapheno-femoral junction commonly referred to as high ligation. This was followed by ligation of the tributaries of the long saphenous vein (there are no tributaries to the femoral vein at this level) followed by stripping of the vein to the knee and multiple avulsions below that if needed. When the vein is stripped in its entirety, there is a risk of damage to the saphenous nerve that runs alongside the vein in the lower leg. Recognition of this fact led to a more limited stripping and local avulsions.

> ### Friedrich Trendelenburg 1844 - 1924
>
> He was a German surgeon who had a great interest in the study of veins and lower limbs.
>
> He described the Trendelenburg position – the head down position which is useful in pelvic surgery.
>
> He also described the Trendelenburg gait as a method of identifying problems with the hip

Short Saphenous Varicosity

For the short saphenous varicosity, the operation is one of ligation of the Sapheno-popliteal junction and avulsions of the distal varicosities in the leg.

Currently, this operation is carried out less and less frequently in the West as more non-invasive methods of sclerosing the veins have become the established norm.

Types of Sclerotherapies

- Chemical
- Mechanical

Chemical Sclerotherapy

This involves the instillation of a salt solution into the vein, causing a chemical reaction in the walls of the veins. This has been in practice since the 1930s, and the results have been reasonable in selected patients with a satisfactory result in up 80 per cent of treated patients. Not all patients will be suitable for this. It is contraindicated in pregnant women; it must be used with caution in patients on oral contraceptives. In patients with a cardiac history who may need a bypass in the future, the exclusion of these veins that are used in bypass surgery will need cautious evaluation.

A modern variation of this technique is foam sclerotherapy, where air is added to the chemical solution resulting in an equally satisfactory result with less discomfort.

These procedures involve the instillation of the chemical solution into the vein or into spider veins. The veins are emptied, and the chemical is instilled. A compression crepe bandage is applied to approximate the opposing walls of the vein that become inflamed following the chemical irritation. The vein walls adhere, and the vein collapses as a result and is excluded from circulation.

Mechanical Sclerotherapy

- Endothermal ablation
- Laser ablation
- Glue ablation

The principle here is similar to chemical sclerotherapy, but the procedure is done under ultrasound guidance. Local, regional, or general anaesthesia may be appropriate. The vein is cannulated at the ankle or knee, and an endothermal or laser probe is passed up to the sapheno-femoral or sapheno-popliteal junction. The location is confirmed with ultrasound. As the probe is withdrawn it is activated. The local heat causes a reconfiguration of the protein in the walls and causes them to adhere, effectively excluding the vein from further circulation. This has the same effect as stripping. Long-term studies have shown a very low recannulation rate. Glue injections work similarly by obliterating the veins and are still being evaluated.

CHOLECYSTITIS AND BILIARY DISEASE

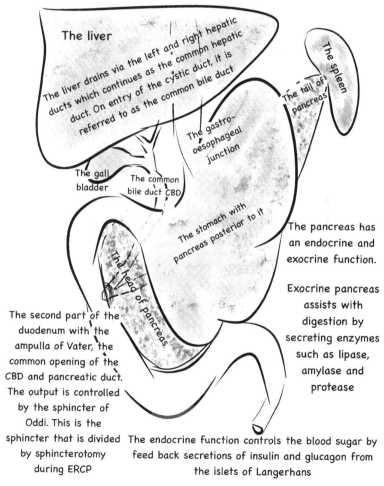

The liver

The liver drains via the left and right hepatic ducts which continues as the common hepatic duct. On entry of the cystic duct, it is referred to as the common bile duct

The spleen

The tail of pancreas

The gastro-oesophageal junction

The gall bladder

The common bile duct CBD

The stomach with pancreas posterior to it

The head of pancreas

The second part of the duodenum with the ampulla of Vater, the common opening of the CBD and pancreatic duct. The output is controlled by the sphincter of Oddi. This is the sphincter that is divided by sphincterotomy during ERCP

The pancreas has an endocrine and exocrine function.

Exocrine pancreas assists with digestion by secreting enzymes such as lipase, amylase and protease

The endocrine function controls the blood sugar by feed back secretions of insulin and glucagon from the islets of Langerhans

Figure 14: Hepatobiliary tree and pancreas

79

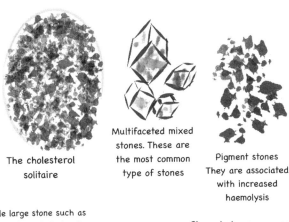

The cholesterol
solitaire

Multifaceted mixed
stones. These are
the most common
type of stones

Pigment stones
They are associated
with increased
haemolysis

Single large stone such as
the solitary cholesterol
stone can block the cystic
duct causing a mucocoele
of the gall bladder

Pigment stones may occur
with Thalassaemia, sickle
cell disease and other
congenital conditions that
cause increased
haemolysis.

Figure 15: Types of gall stones

1. Gallstones are caused by an imbalance between bile salts, cholesterol, and lecithin leading to super saturation and crystallisation.
2. Cholesterol stones may be due to dietary factors; loss of bile salts due to terminal ileal resection (where bile salts are absorbed), and the contraceptive pill.
3. Pigment stones (the pigment is bilirubin related salt) arise due to acquired or congenital haemolytic anaemia (hereditary spherocytosis); metallic cardiac valve replacements may lead to crunching of the RBCs with each beat causing haemolysis, sickle cell disease, and even thalassaemia.
4. Mixed stones are a combination of cholesterol and pigment. These are the most common. Typically, one is likely to see a single large cholesterol stone at the cystic duct with a brood of multifaceted mix stones filling the gall bladder.
5. The stones may be asymptomatic.
6. Symptoms can arise from stones within the gallbladder when they can cause:
    *   Acute cholecystitis
    *   Biliary colic

- Chronic cholecystitis
- Mucocoele of the gallbladder due to blockage of cystic duct
- Empyema when such a blockage gets infected
- Perforation of the gall bladder, leading to bile peritonitis
7. If the stones slip into the common bile duct, they can cause
   - jaundice due to blockage of the duct and
   - pancreatitis when they block the common channel of the pancreatic and bile ducts at the ampulla of Vater.
8. In some situations, they can cause a fistula between the gallbladder and duodenum, and stones may slip out into the small bowel and cause gallstone ileus when they get impacted in the ileum, where the lumen may be narrower than the jejunum.
9. Treatment such as cholecystectomy may be necessary to prevent complications arising.

Cholecystitis and biliary colic are common problems due to stones in the gall bladder. Traditionally it is said to affect 'the fat, fertile female of forty'. This is no longer the case as society is changing. Younger people on contraceptives present earlier.

The majority of people with gallstones have little or no symptoms. Biliary colic and cholecystitis are the commonest, with less than 2 per cent presenting with the dreaded complication of pancreatitis.

About 20 per cent of people over sixty years of age will have gallstones on imaging with ultrasound scan but may not have symptoms.

Acute Presentation

Acute cholecystitis is one of the most common conditions that need emergency admissions. Most patients present with pain in the right upper quadrant of the abdomen; this may follow a fatty meal, but not exclusively. Some patients will have had a similar but milder pain after food that they had overlooked for many months or even years.

The pain is typically brought on by eating fatty foods and is located in the right upper quadrant of the abdomen. The gallbladder is a foregut derivative, and hence the pain can also present in the epigastric region and rarely in the retrosternal region, mimicking a myocardial event.

Acute cholecystitis presents with constant pain, and the patient may have pyrexia. Tenderness may be present in the right upper quadrant.

Murphy's sign may be positive; this is demonstrated by palpating the right upper quadrant of the abdomen. The fundus of the gallbladder is located at the tip of the right ninth costal cartilage in the trans-pyloric plane. An inflamed gallbladder is therefore directly under the tip of the ninth costal cartilage. The palpating hand is placed under the costal cartilage in the right upper quadrant of the abdomen. The patient is asked to take a deep breath, and as the diaphragmatic movement pushes the liver and gallbladder inferiorly, the inflamed gallbladder is pressed against the palpating hand. This causes the patient to catch the breath as the fundus of the inflamed gallbladder hits the palpating hand.

It is important to distinguish biliary colic from acute cholecystitis. Biliary colic is a misnomer. Typically, it is not a colic and lasts from a few minutes to a few hours. It settles down as quickly as it starts. It may occur due to a temporary obstruction of the cystic duct due to tiny mobile stones that are pushed out by contraction of the gallbladder after a fatty meal. The stones fall back into the gallbladder with the relaxation of the gallbladder, and the pain resolves. White cell count may be normal.

Berkeley Moynihan 1865 -1936

He described the Murphy's sign of pain on deep inspiration.

I have found the simplest method of eliciting the pressure signs to be this: While the surgeon sits on the edge of the couch, to the right of the patient, the left hand is laid over the lower part of the right side of the patient's chest, so that the thumb lies along the rib-margin; as a deep breath is taken the thumb is pressed upwards towards the under surface of the liver.

He was considered an authority on abdominal surgery and was President of the Royal College of Surgeons. He is known to have stated 'every gall stone is a tombstone erected to the memory of dead bacteria'. We now know that the process of formation is chemical and not infective although infection may supervene at a later stage, the stones are not due to infection. They can cause *infections*.

*'The scalpel is, indeed, an instrument of most precious use – in some hands a royal sceptre; in others but a rude mattock. The perfect surgeon must have the 'heart of a lion and the hand of a lady'; never the claws of a lion and the heart of a sheep. **An operation is done quick enough when it is done right'. Moynihan 1913.***

This is true even today!

The following predisposing factors may be absent but are noteworthy.

- Weight gain
- Rapid weight loss
- Recent pregnancy: bile stasis can lead to formation of stones
- Oral contraceptives
- Crohn's disease: absence of absorption of bile salts in the distal ileum may lead to an imbalance and precipitate stone formation; this may follow ileal resection or bypass
- Aortic valve replacement with mechanical valve
- Haemolytic anaemia

Haemolytic anaemia can be hereditary or acquired. Once RBCs lose their biconcave shape and become rounded as in hereditary spherocytosis, they are easily broken down in the spleen. Drugs and metallic valve replacements may cause haemolysis. Haemolysis leads to an excess of bile pigments and thus to stone formation

Family history is not of significance, but there are families with lithogenic bile. The most common reason for a strong family history is that the families are brought up eating and enjoying similar types of food.

Investigations

The rules to follow for investigations are constant for all diseases. Here they are in order:

- Urine
- Blood
- Radiology
- Others

Urine

Dip stick for sugar, protein, blood, bilirubin, urobilinogen, and nitrates. In young women, beta HCG is very important. If coincidentally positive, you may not want any radiological imaging with X-rays. Nitrates if positive will suggest incidental urinary infections; likewise, with a raised sugar and diabetes.

Blood

Full blood count (FBC), CRP, urea, electrolytes, liver function test, and serum amylase are very basic in all patients. The white cell count and CRP may be raised if there is acute cholecystitis and may be normal in biliary colic.

Radiology

An X-ray of the chest or abdomen is unnecessary if the patient is not suspected of having an acute abdomen; 90 per cent of gall stones are not radio opaque. (note: 90 per cent of renal stones that are radio opaque).

An ultrasound examination of the abdomen in most cases will confirm the diagnosis; in the very obese, the bodily habitus will make the ultrasound examination difficult, and a CT or MRI will be needed. A CT scan, however, is not as good as an ultrasound examination in picking up stones in the gallbladder.

Other investigations:

MRI of the liver and gallbladder may be needed if the ultrasound findings are equivocal.

A HIDA scan is used for an assessment of the physiological function of the gallbladder. This will assess the emptying time of the gallbladder after a fatty meal. When the test is positive, the gallbladder will show delayed emptying after a fatty meal. It can also possibly be caused by a small stone blocking the cystic duct in the valves (valve of Heister) that represent mucosal folds in the cystic duct. This is by no means proven.

Magnetic resonance cholangio-pancreatography (MRCP) is done when there is a biochemically elevated serum bilirubin. This will define the calibre of the common duct and the presence of pathology in the duct. It may demonstrate the presence of stones in the gall bladder or CBD and the need for invasive intervention such as an endoscopic retrograde cholangio-pancreatography (ERCP). The present policy is therefore to do this as a screening procedure prior to the more invasive ERCP.

Management

The diagnosis of biliary colic may enable a laparoscopic cholecystectomy on that admission. Patients presenting with acute cholecystitis must also be operated upon on the same admission if fit for surgery. In the presence of cholecystitis there is a higher conversion rate from a laparoscopic to an open operation. The advantage of an early operation is the ability to provide a curative treatment that will avoid complications during the waiting period. Equally, the diagnostic facilities now allow for early operation compared to the times when patients were placed on a waiting list and brought in for interval cholecystectomy much later.

When a patient is symptomatic from gallstones, then surgical treatment will merit consideration. Much depends on the suitability of the patient for surgery and the absence of comorbidity. As always in all of surgery, the decision to operate is a fine balance between the perceived benefits and risk of surgery. Safety in selection of patients leads to safety in surgery.

Recall the oft repeated statement "The feasibility of an operation is never an indication for its performance' (Henry Ogilvie).

Courvoisier's Law

In the 1880's Ludwig Georg Courvoisier observed that in a jaundiced patient with a painless palpable gallbladder, gallstones were an unlikely cause. He did not suggest carcinoma of the pancreas. He did not call it a law. He did not state the exceptions now recognised, of a double duct impaction with a blocked cystic duct and a blocked common bile duct.

Mirizzi Syndrome

In this rare syndrome, a stone in the neck of the cystic duct blocks the common bile duct as well, thereby causing jaundice as well as a palpable gallbladder.

SURGICAL JAUNDICE

In pre hepatic jaundice there is an increase in the level of unconjugated bilirubin. This may be secondary to production of bilirubin that exceeds the capacity of the hepatocyte to process it. This type of jaundice is represented by the Gilbert's syndrome a congenital disorder due to an inborn error of metabolism

Pre Hepatic Jaundice

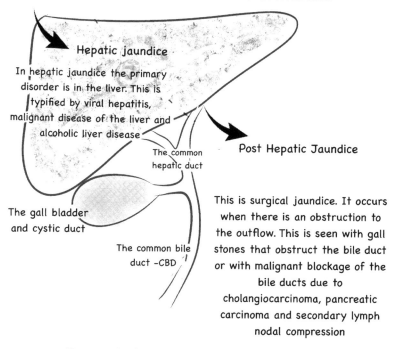

Hepatic jaundice

In hepatic jaundice the primary disorder is in the liver. This is typified by viral hepatitis, malignant disease of the liver and alcoholic liver disease

The common hepatic duct

Post Hepatic Jaundice

The gall bladder and cystic duct

The common bile duct -CBD

This is surgical jaundice. It occurs when there is an obstruction to the outflow. This is seen with gall stones that obstruct the bile duct or with malignant blockage of the bile ducts due to cholangiocarcinoma, pancreatic carcinoma and secondary lymph nodal compression

Figure 16: Showing types of jaundice

Types of Jaundice:

- **Pre-hepatic**
- **Hepatic**
- **Post-hepatic**

Jaundice occurs secondary to elevated products of haemoglobin metabolism due to several factors. The hepatocytes in the liver process the waste products of haem.

Typically, the classification is based on the location of the hold up and thus it can be pre-hepatic, hepatic, or post-hepatic. Surgical jaundice is commonly post-hepatic due to outlet obstruction.

Pathophysiology

- RBC is broken down in the spleen/liver/marrow
- Haemoglobin is split into haem and globin
- Globin and iron from haem are recycled
- The rest of the haem is broken down to biliverdin and then to bilirubin, which assists in production of bile that is needed to emulsify dietary fat

Step 1: The unconjugated bilirubin is fat soluble and thus is transported with albumin to the liver.

Step 2: The bilirubin is then conjugated in the hepatocyte with glucuronic acid, which renders it water soluble.

Step 3: The conjugated water-soluble bilirubin is excreted into the biliary duct system and enters the duodenum. There it is broken down by bacterial action, a process that occurs in the intestines, which removes and recycles the glucuronic acid. The bilirubin that remains is converted to stercobilinogen. It is the stercobilinogen that gives the colour to stools. The bilirubin that is absorbed into the blood stream is urobilinogen and is excreted in urine.

It stands to reason that when the urobilinogen is absent in the urine in a jaundiced patient, there must be an obstruction to the outflow from liver. With reappearance of urobilinogen in the urine the obstruction is deemed to have cleared. In the days prior to ultrasonography, a urobilinogen chart at the bedside in jaundiced patients indicating reappearance of urobilinogen in the urine heralded the passage of stones in the common bile duct.

If a patient presents with jaundice that is noted to be secondary to a dilated common bile duct noted on ultrasound or CT scan, then the causes are likely to be surgical.

Normally the common bile duct has a diameter of 6 mm in the absence of previous interventional procedures such as ERCP. As the common duct has no smooth muscle, once it has become dilated, it will stay dilated always. If the CBD is dilated and the patient is jaundiced, the next step is to define the cause of obstruction. A MRCP is done as a first step prior to an interventional ERCP.

In an acute presentation with jaundice, the cause is likely to be stones in the common bile duct, especially when a gallbladder is not palpable. (Curuvoisier)

Other causes are malignancies of the pancreas or the common bile duct, sclerosing cholangitis, and benign strictures of the CBD.

If CBD stones are diagnosed, the patient will need to be referred for ERCP for extraction of the stone. A sphincterotomy (division of the sphincter of Oddi at the ampulla of Vater) may be needed for removal of the calculus with or without the placement of a stent.

Causes of Surgical Jaundice

- Stones in the common bile duct
- Carcinoma of the head of the pancreas
- Peri-ampullary carcinoma
- Malignancies in the liver

- Pancreatitis
- Cholangio carcinoma
- Secondaries around the hepatic ducts
- Sclerosing cholangitis
- Strictures of the common bile duct

PANCREATITIS

Pancreatic inflammation can be acute or chronic. The presentations are very different. Acute pancreatitis is a life-threatening disease. Chronic pancreatitis presents entirely differently and will not be discussed here other than to highlight the different presentation at the end of the chapter.

The revised Atlanta classification requires that two or more of the following criteria be met for the diagnosis of acute pancreatitis.

1. Abdominal pain suggestive of pancreatitis
2. Serum amylase or lipase level greater than three times the upper normal value
3. Characteristic imaging findings on CT or MRI (P. A. Banks, T. L. Bollen, C. Dervenis, et al., 'Classification of Acute Pancreatitis 2012: Revision of the Atlanta Classification and Definitions by International Consensus', *Gut* 62, no. 1 [2013]: 102–11)

Acute Pancreatitis Presentation

- Sudden onset of abdominal pain
- Vomiting is almost always present
- Tachycardia
- Tenderness localised in epigastrium or generalised all over the four quadrants with peritonitis
- Temperature with pyrexia greater than 38 degrees Celsius
- Known history of high alcohol intake
- Known history of gall stones, a common cause

- Elevated inflammatory markers
- Elevated serum amylase or lipase

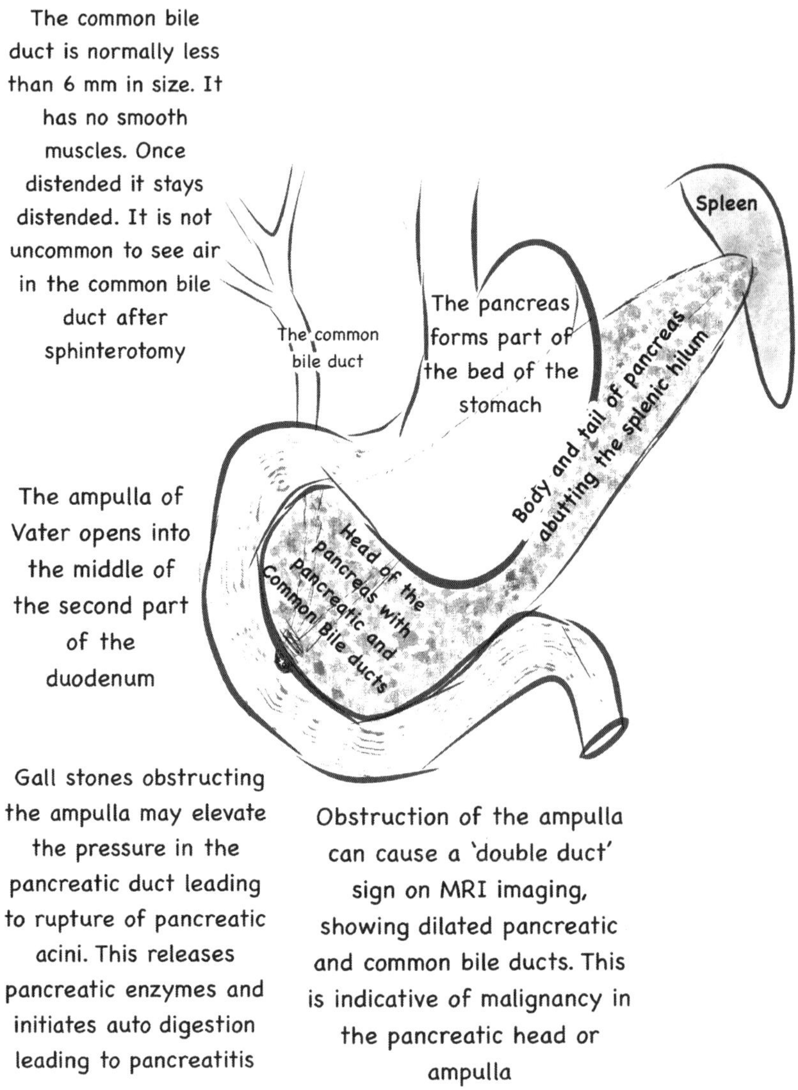

The common bile duct is normally less than 6 mm in size. It has no smooth muscles. Once distended it stays distended. It is not uncommon to see air in the common bile duct after sphinterotomy

The common bile duct

The pancreas forms part of the bed of the stomach

Spleen

Body and tail of pancreas abutting the splenic hilum

Head of the pancreas with pancreatic and Common Bile ducts

The ampulla of Vater opens into the middle of the second part of the duodenum

Gall stones obstructing the ampulla may elevate the pressure in the pancreatic duct leading to rupture of pancreatic acini. This releases pancreatic enzymes and initiates auto digestion leading to pancreatitis

Obstruction of the ampulla can cause a 'double duct' sign on MRI imaging, showing dilated pancreatic and common bile ducts. This is indicative of malignancy in the pancreatic head or ampulla

Figure 17: Anatomy and physiology of the pancreas

Pathophysiology

Although hidden in the retroperitoneum behind the stomach, the pancreas is a major player in the control of blood sugar and digestion. It has a very significant endocrine and exocrine function.

The endocrine function plays a big role in the management of sugar by way of the hormones insulin and glucagon. The exocrine function plays a functional role by secreting enzymes such as amylase, protease, and lipase. Amylase digests carbohydrate to glucose; protease digests proteins to amino acids, and lipase digests fats to fatty acids. The enzymes amylase and lipase are markers for inflammation of the pancreas. These enzymes do not digest the pancreas because they are secreted as proenzymes that are broken down in the alkaline succus entericus or enteric fluid in the duodenum. If the acini in which they are secreted is breached as in pancreatitis, they then digest the pancreas by a process of auto-digestion. An increase in the intra-acinar pressure leads to rupture of the acini, leading to pancreatic auto-digestion, inflammation, and pancreatitis. It is postulated that gallstones that block the pancreatic duct can increase the back pressure on the main pancreatic duct acutely, leading to rupture and release of enzymes. Much as gravel in a jar does not block the flow of water (filtration of drinking water depends on this), stones in the common bile duct will allow flow of bile down the duct unless it is blocked at the outlet at the ampulla of Vater. The exact mechanism by which alcohol does that is still not clear, but spasm of the sphincter of Oddi around the ampulla leading to obstruction may be a factor.

Fatty food in the duodenum causes the production of cholecystokinin-pancreozymin (CCK-PZ) that makes the gallbladder contract and release bile to enable breakdown of fat in the food to micelles and facilitate its absorption. The liver also releases bile, but the gallbladder contraction leads to a surge of bile to help digest the icing on the cake that is eaten. This process can lead to small stones being pushed down the common bile duct, leading to jaundice and, in some unlucky patients, pancreatitis. Jaundice does not always accompany pancreatitis. It is presumed the stones, after causing the pancreatitis, have passed into the intestines after a transient blockage. Still, the commonest causes are gallstones and alcohol intake (not dose dependent). If they are excluded, then rarer causes need to be sought.

Causes of Acute Pancreatitis

- Gall stones
- Alcohol intake
- Post ERCP
- Hypercalcaemia or Hyperlipidaemia
- Microlithiasis in pancreatic duct
- Autoimmune pancreatitis
- Ampullary or pancreatic tumours
- Anatomical anomalies (pancreas divisum)

Note: Common things are commoner and rare things rarer

Serum Amylase

When serum amylase is elevated to three times the normal value, a diagnosis of pancreatitis is most likely in conjunction with clinical findings and clinical diagnosis. The serum amylase may be raised in other conditions too, and it is non-specific. In acute pancreatitis, the level rises rapidly and falls rapidly. Serum amylase may thus not be elevated if the patient presents late. In those circumstances, serum lipase is a useful marker because it stays elevated for longer after an acute attack.

Serum Amylase:

- Rises within 3 hrs and decreases in 3 days
- Any peritoneal inflammation can cause elevation of amylase (Peritonitis)
- Increased amylase with abdominal symptoms is seen in:
  - Ectopic pregnancy
  - Post ERCP
  - Peptic perforation
  - Ischaemic bowel
- Other causes without abdominal symptoms:
  - Congenital hyperamylasaemia
  - Chronic alcoholism
  - Liver failure

Once diagnosed as acute pancreatitis, the management is primarily non-operative. At presentation, it is difficult to predict the course of the disease. A small proportion of patients deteriorate and are a likely to need management at a level of care higher than that of the ward, possibly in a critical care unit.

There are a number of parameters that can be used to predict the severity of the disease over the first forty-eight hours. A commonly used measure is the Ranson's criteria.

In some patients presenting with severe haemorrhagic pancreatitis, there can be visible evidence of haemorrhage in the form of bruising around the umbilicus (Cullen's sign). The blood from the retroperitoneum seems to track via either the falciform ligament or the mid-umbilical ligament along the attachment of the urachus.

In rare cases, similar bruising can be seen in the flanks and is referred to as the Grey Turner's sign.

Ranson's Criteria

- Age above than 55 years
- White cell count above 15 x109/ L
- Blood glucose above 10 mmol/L (non-diabetic)
- LDH above 600 IU/L
- AST above 200 u/L
- Corrected calcium less than 2.0 mmol/L
- Blood urea above 16 mmol/L (Normal previously)
- Arterial pO2 less than 8 kPa (60 mm Hg)
- Metabolic acidosis
- Decreasing haematocrit after 48 hrs

- **Serum amylase is not an indicator of severity**

Positive Criteria and Mortality

0-2	<5% mortality
3-4	20% mortality
5-6	40% mortality
7-8	100% mortality

Respiratory problems such as ARDS arise due to digestion of surfactant, a mucopolysaccharide that keeps open the alveoli due to surface tension. This may occur due to the action of pancreatic enzymes that leak into the thorax. Once the surfactant is decreased, the alveoli collapse, causing a shunt due to a ventilation, perfusion mismatch. The compliance of the lung decreases, the lungs stiffen, and patients are then likely to drop their O_2 saturation despite adequate delivery of oxygen. It may progress to lung injury with a need for ventilation and possibly positive pressure ventilation.

Calcium levels can drop due to the release of lipase that digests fat to glycerol and fatty acids as the end products of fat digestion. The fatty acids will then react with calcium to form soap. This process is referred to as saponification of fat. At operations for pancreatitis (rare these days), fat necrosis of the omentum can be visible. Current management makes laparotomies very unlikely, and this finding will probably be relegated to history, although it is good to know of a possible cause for low calcium levels in pancreatitis. It is likely to be multifactorial, however, and also involves effects secondary to a drop in albumin levels (Imrie 1978) and refractoriness to parathormone.

Management

The principles of management are the same as for all acute presentations, as discussed earlier. Specifics of management for acute pancreatitis involve confirmation of suspicion that the patient has pancreatitis, noting the baseline severity and providing supportive treatment under constant scrutiny in a HDU-level environment.

Principles of Management

Immediate assessment: ABCDE
Never forget pulse oximetry

Immediate investigations
- Urine for nitrates, beta-hcg, sugar and blood
- Blood for sugar, full blood count, electrolytes and urea, coagulation profile
- Radiology
- Comorbidity assessment: Acute myocardial event, diabetes, COPD, Renal status and Anti-coagulants

Specific management for pancreatitis
Serum amylase and CRP
Baseline blood gas and monitoring of oxygen saturation
Liver function tests
CT scan is best done after 3 to 4 days as the criteria are best established later than at outset.
MRCP followed by ERCP in the presence of Jaundice
Coagulation profile prior to ERCP
Attention to nutrition. No need to restrict fluids and diet unless the patient is unable to retain oral fluids
No indication for routine antibiotics as the problem is initially chemical than infective but needs careful monitoring

The SILDA Mantra

Stabilisation: Blood pressure over 90mmhg/O2 >94%
Investigation: Concurrently with making the patient stable
Localisation: Find the cause
Decision: Type of care- conservative, interventional, palliative
Action: Prompt action saves lives. No vacillation

Early treatment is limited to assessment, monitoring, and maintaining fluid balance along with adequate analgesia and oxygenation, and oral fluids as tolerated. Nasogastric tube is seldom needed unless the patient has ongoing vomiting. Antibiotics are not introduced early but may be needed if there is evidence of necrosis on CT.

CT Severity index - Balthazar	
Assessment of inflammation of pancreas	
No Inflammation	0
Focal or diffuse enlargement	1
Peripancreatic inflammation	2
Single ill-defined fluid collection/Phlegmon	3
Two or more ill-defined collections/peripancreatic gas	4
Pancreatic necrosis	
None	0
1/3 necrosis or less	2
1/2 necrosis	4
Greater than 1/2 necrosis	6
The severity is then calculated based on the score	

If the patient deteriorates, the level of support will increase. In the UK, it is necessary to discuss further care in a specialist hepato-biliary unit. A transfer to the unit may be necessary if further interventions are required.

Ventilation with PEEP, ERCP to remove obstruction at the level of the ampulla, radiological or surgical drainage, and necrosectomy (either open or minimally invasive) may be needed.

Multi-organ failure is a major problem. Antibiotics will then be dictated by culture of blood, sputum or intra-abdominal aspirate especially in the presence of infected necrosis and chest infections.

Pancreatic abscess can form secondary to necrosis. This complication arises within the first two to three weeks, unlike a pseudocyst that manifests later.

Pancreatic pseudo-cysts are cysts that arise in the peri-pancreatic tissue. They are referred to as pseudo-cysts because they are not lined by epithelium, as true cysts are, but by mesothelial structures surrounding the pancreas that wall off collections. Yet some of these cysts may communicate with the pancreatic duct, and when they do, most resolve over time. If the cysts fail to resolve after six weeks to three months, then they can be drained endoscopically through a cysto-gastrostomy. In general, the procedure is safe to perform when the cyst wall shows evidence of being mature and well defined. Some cysts may not be accessible for this non-invasive procedure and may need radiological or surgical drainage.

Greater than one-third of patients tend to have mild pancreatitis. When the pancreatitis is secondary to gallstones, then a cholecystectomy is recommended within two weeks of the acute episode, and preferably in the same admission subject to comorbidities and other limitations. This can be a technically challenging procedure in the early days.

Complications of Pancreatitis

- Pancreatic abscess – This occurs after two or more weeks
- Pancreatic Pseudocyst
- Pancreatic fistula
- Pancreatic insufficiency
- Diabetes
- Chronic pancreatitis

Chronic Pancreatitis

This presents with symptoms that are very different to that of the acute episode. Chronic pain can be disabling and needs to be addressed by a multidisciplinary team involving the gastroenterologists and pain team.

Chronic Pancreatitis Presentation

- **Diabetes:** loss of endocrine pancreatic function
- **Diarrhoea:** Due to loss of exocrine function
- **Chronic pain:** Neuropathic secondary to chronic inflammation of retroperitoneum

BOWEL OBSTRUCTION

Acute presentation with obstruction to the large or small bowel is a common cause for admission to the hospital.

Four Pillars of Presentation of Bowel Obstruction

- Constipation or obstipation (not passing stools and flatus)
- Abdominal distension
- Abdominal pain
- Vomiting

The presentation tends to vary depending on the level of obstruction. The lower the obstruction, the more likely that the patient will present with all the four signs and symptoms. It stands to reason that the higher the obstruction, the more likely that vomiting will be the predominant feature rather than distension or constipation.

Common Causes of Bowel Obstruction

- Adhesive bowel obstruction
- Hernial obstruction
- Malignant bowel obstruction
- Post-operative or paralytic ileus
- Ischaemic and inflammatory bowel disease
- Bands causing obstruction
- Volvulus of caecum or sigmoid

- Internal herniation
- Radiation strictures
- Foreign body causing obstruction
- Gall stone ileus
- Pseudo-obstruction
- Perforated viscus and peritonitis
- Inflammatory bowel disease

Adhesive bowel obstruction is perhaps the most common cause of acute obstruction of the bowel. It usually follows previous laparotomies. Most patients will have a scar of an abdominal incision, though sometimes with the passage of time, the scars in the groin or supra pubic area may not be clearly visible.

Adhesive obstructions due to bands do occur but are less frequent.

A hernia of one type or another, but more commonly a femoral or inguinal hernia, can cause bowel obstruction. Incisional and para-umbilical hernia may also present as acute obstruction. In most of these presentations, the hernia will be clearly visible. In some patients, it may have been irreducible for a considerable length of time. In the elderly patients, a superficial examination of the abdomen may entirely miss the presence of a femoral hernia. The dictum 'No examination of the abdomen is complete unless the groin and genitalia are examined' is one that must be put to practice in all acutely admitted patients with abdominal symptoms.

Malignancies of the colon and small bowel can cause bowel obstruction depending on the location of the tumour. In the case of the right colonic cancers, it is the caecum or ascending colon that is the source of the blockage, and it will present with small bowel obstruction. A malignant tumour in the left colon and distal colon cancers are more likely to cause colonic obstruction.

Sigmoid volvulus is a condition where the sigmoid colon tends to rotate in an anticlockwise direction around a mesentery that has become elongated over time. The mesenteric base of attachment to the abdominal wall is narrow. A narrow and fixed base with an elongated mesentery facilitates rotation around the fixed point. It is common in elderly patients and in patients in long-term care and those on psychiatric medications. The presentation is one of large bowel obstruction.

Caecal volvulus is uncommon but occurs in the presence of a mobile caecum that is not fixed to the retroperitoneum. The caecum in these conditions will be noted in the left upper quadrant on imaging associated with small bowel obstruction. It can also follow congenital malrotation or congenital Ladd's bands associated with malrotation.

Diverticular stenosis and extrinsic pelvic pathology can also present with obstruction.

Inflammatory bowel disease such as Crohn's and ulcerative colitis may present with obstruction; these are now more common after failed response to primary medical management. Patients with Crohn's disease are prone to multiple stricture formation in the bowel.

Pseudo-obstruction of the colon is another uncommon presentation. In this condition, the colon and small bowel in the presence of an incontinent ileocaecal valve appear distended but without a definable mechanical obstruction.

As the name implies, paralytic ileus is an obstruction due to the loss of normal motility of the bowel. It generally occurs in the post-operative period due to electrolyte or protein imbalance. In patients with low albumin, the bowel wall becomes oedematous, and the peristaltic process is impeded.

Principles of Management

Immediate assessment: ABCDE
> Never forget pulse oximetry

Immediate investigations:
- Urine for nitrates, beta-hcg, sugar and blood
- Blood for sugar, full blood count, electrolytes and urea, coagulation profile
- **Radiology**

Comorbidity assessment
- ECG to exclude acute myocardial event
- Diabetes
- COPD
- Renal status
- Use of anti-coagulants

Call for Assistance/Allied speciality advice

Specific to bowel obstruction

Naso-gastric decompression in cases with persistent vomiting

Intravenous fluid replacement

Monitoring of intake and output

Radiology for assisting assessment and diagnosis including Erect chest x-ray, Supine x-ray of the abdomen and CT scan

Gastrograffin or soluble oral contrast imaging of bowel

The SILDA Mantra

Stabilisation: Blood pressure over 90mmhg/O2 >94%

Investigation: Concurrently with making the patient stable

Localisation: Find the cause

Decision: Type of care- conservative, interventional, palliative

Action: Prompt action saves lives. No vacillation

Management follows the same protocols, as seen earlier.

The supine X-rays of the abdomen will be able to define the level of obstruction, but this is increasingly supplanted by CT scan as the main radiological investigation because it can suggest not only the level of obstruction but also the cause of obstruction.

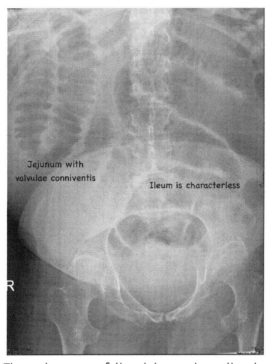

The supine x-ray of the abdomen shows the clear pattern of an obstructed jejunum with valvulae conniventis that run fully across the bowel unlike colonic haustra that outline only across part ot the width of the bowel. The ileum being thin walled is characterless

Figure 18: Pattern seen in small bowel obstruction

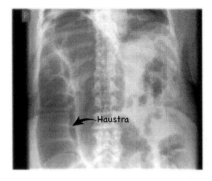

The pattern of colonic mucosa on x-rays is different from that of the jejunum. The mucosal fold lines unlike that of the jejunum, do not go fully across the width of the bowel but stop short of touching the opposite wall. These are called haustra

In these x-rays, the haustra are seen clearly. This patient had a volvulus

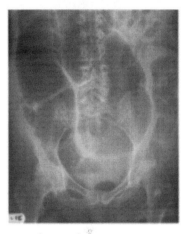

Figure 19: Pattern seen in colonic obstruction

Once the diagnosis is confirmed, the treatment is directed towards either interventional surgical management or non-interventional but active medical management. The latter may be needed due to comorbidities and rests on the fitness of the patient to undergo major interventional surgery. A wait and watch policy may be adopted in patients with adhesive obstruction because recurrent surgical operations may cause more harm, however surgical intervention is likely to be needed if the obstruction fails to resolve soon and the patient is fit for surgery. Prolonged obstruction without resolution leads to associated complications with nutrition and metabolism. Sometimes surgical intervention is inevitable, as in patients presenting with evidence of ischaemia, strangulation, or perforation leading to peritonitis. These may be clinically evident with generalised tenderness or peritonitis. A raised WBC and CRP should alert one to the possibility of impending bowel ischaemia or strangulation.

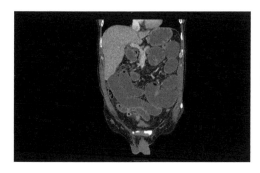

These CT scans show clear evidence of small bowel obstruction. The advantage of a CT over a plain X-ray is that whilst confirming obstruction it is also likely to indicate the cause and the level at which the obstruction occurs

The distended loops of jejunum with valvulae conniventis that resemble the steps of a ladder are clearly seen on these scans. The jejunum is fluid loaded and obstructed

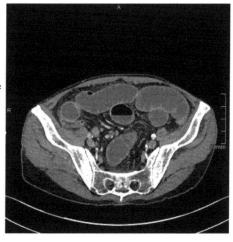

CT scans will eventually obviate the need for a plain x-ray of the abdomen. They are proving to be a most useful tool in surgical management based on the principle ' investigate before intervention'

Figure 20: CT scan showing small bowel obstruction

Where there is evidence of adhesive bowel obstruction without ischaemia or strangulation, a wait and watch policy is justified. Gastrograffin or soluble oral contrast swallow is used to assess the feasibility of non-operative management. The gastrograffin contains 'tween 80', and this can decrease the oedema in the bowel wall, leading to relief of obstruction demonstrated by progression of gastrograffin to the distal bowel beyond the area of obstruction. In many patients with adhesive small bowel obstruction, this can be used as a radiological test of suitability for conservative management with the ultimate goal of resolution of obstruction without intervention. Regular and repeated assessments are needed if a non-operative management is followed. The management, though not interventional, is active and includes twice daily review of the patient till a satisfactory outcome is reached.

In colonic obstruction due to left-sided malignancies of the colon, the area of tenderness may be located over the caecum. Caecum is the thinnest part of the colon that has the maximal diameter. In colonic obstruction in the distal or left colon, as the wall of the caecum is thinner, it tends to distend early and more rapidly than the rest of the colon. Laplace stated that the pressure on the wall is greatest where the radius is largest. The caecum, being the widest and thinnest, is the easiest to distend with increasing pressure. Progressive distention causes ischaemia due to stretching and may lead to caecal perforation. This distension is maximal if the ileo-caecal valve is competent. When the valve is incompetent, the presentation may involve small bowel obstruction. On radiological imaging, if the caecum is distended beyond 12 cm, it should raise suspicion of impending ischaemia or caecal perforation.

Pseudo-obstruction of the colon is exactly what it means. There is obstruction of the bowel but no recognisable mechanical cause. This is common in institutionalised patients and those with serious underlying electrolyte and metabolic irregularities. If accompanied by perforation, the mortality rate can be high. A similar presentation occurs in volvulus of the sigmoid.

Management follows the same standard principles outlined earlier. If a laparotomy is undertaken, then resection of bowel and primary anastomosis or release of adhesions with resolution of the obstruction should be feasible. Generalised faecal or purulent peritonitis may dictate the need for a stoma of one form or another with drainage of the peritoneal cavity. Colonic malignancies may be resectable with a Hartmann's procedure (discussed in a later chapter).

DIVERTICULAR DISEASE OF THE COLON

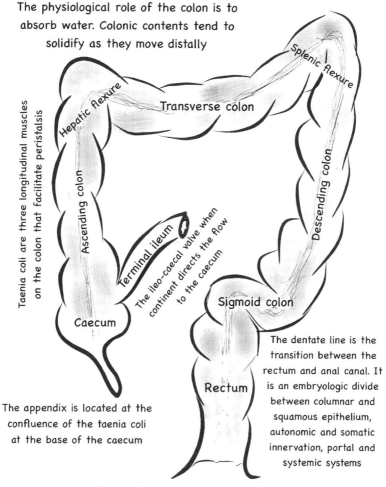

The physiological role of the colon is to absorb water. Colonic contents tend to solidify as they move distally

Splenic flexure

Hepatic flexure

Transverse colon

Taenia coli are three longitudinal muscles on the colon that facilitate peristalsis

Ascending colon

Descending colon

Terminal ileum

The ileo-caecal valve when continent directs the flow to the caecum

Sigmoid colon

Caecum

Rectum

The dentate line is the transition between the rectum and anal canal. It is an embryologic divide between columnar and squamous epithelium, autonomic and somatic innervation, portal and systemic systems

The appendix is located at the confluence of the taenia coli at the base of the caecum

Figure 21: Anatomy of the colon

Diverticulosis commonly affects the sigmoid colon but can affect any part or all the colon.

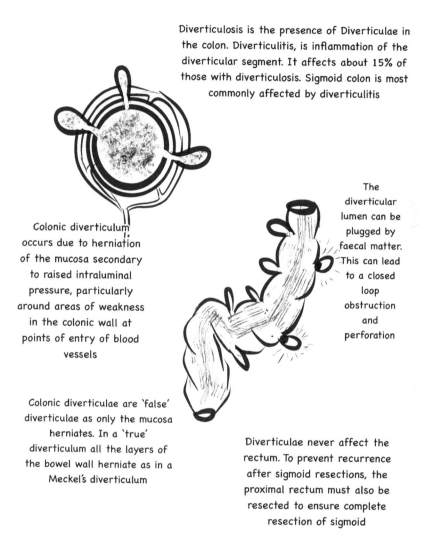

Diverticulosis is the presence of Diverticulae in the colon. Diverticulitis, is inflammation of the diverticular segment. It affects about 15% of those with diverticulosis. Sigmoid colon is most commonly affected by diverticulitis

Colonic diverticulum occurs due to herniation of the mucosa secondary to raised intraluminal pressure, particularly around areas of weakness in the colonic wall at points of entry of blood vessels

The diverticular lumen can be plugged by faecal matter. This can lead to a closed loop obstruction and perforation

Colonic diverticulae are 'false' diverticulae as only the mucosa herniates. In a 'true' diverticulum all the layers of the bowel wall herniate as in a Meckel's diverticulum

Diverticulae never affect the rectum. To prevent recurrence after sigmoid resections, the proximal rectum must also be resected to ensure complete resection of sigmoid

Figure 22: Diverticulosis

Pathophysiology

Diverticula form when the peristaltic pressure in the colon traps a colonic segment full of flatus between succeeding waves, akin to squeezing a balloon at both ends. The bowel has circular muscles and longitudinal muscles.

Circular muscle contraction lengthens the bowel which then goes it to a spasm squeezing the contents. This is followed by the contraction of the longitudinal muscles along with relaxation of the circular muscles. This shortens the bowel and propels the contents. This is a significant force that should not be underestimated. Evolutionarily, it is a similar muscular arrangement that propels the earthworm! This peristaltic force raises the lateral pressure on the walls of the colon and causes herniation of the mucosal lining through areas of weakness at points of entry of the blood vessels into the colon.

Presentation of Diverticulitis

The most common presentation is one of lower abdominal pain that has gradually increased in intensity over a few days. In some it may be an acute presentation.

The signs and symptoms vary depending on the extent of the disease and include the following:

- Abdominal pain, which can be localised to the left lower quadrant of the abdomen
- Tenderness
- Nausea and vomiting
- Pyrexia
- Constipation or, in some patients, looseness of stools
- Occasionally retention of urine with abdominal pain in men
- Excessive vaginal discharge in a few due to colo-vaginal fistula formation
- Passage of flatus in urine or lower urinary tract infection due to colo-vesical fistula
- Peritonitis that is localised to the lower abdomen with pelvic abscess
- Generalised peritonitis
- Bowel obstruction due to diverticular stricture

On admission, the usual protocol that is outlined for all acute admissions should be put into place as per the common generic chart.

Principles of Management

Immediate assessment: ABCDE
>   Never forget pulse oximetry

Immediate investigations:
*   Urine for nitrates, beta-hcg, sugar and blood
*   Blood for sugar, full blood count, electrolytes and urea, coagulation profile
*   **Radiology**

Comorbidity assessment
*   ECG to exclude acute myocardial event
*   Diabetes
*   COPD
*   Renal status
*   Use of anti-coagulants

Call for Assistance/Allied speciality advice

Specific to Diverticulitis
*   CT scan of the abdomen to stage diverticulitis
*   MRI may be needed to define the presence of fistula to vagina, bladder, or small bowel
*   Colonoscopy to view the mucosal aspect and exclude the presence of polyps that may be coincidentally present

The SILDA Mantra

Stabilisation: Blood pressure over 90mmhg/O2 >94%

Investigation: Concurrently with making the patient stable

Localisation: Find the cause

Decision: Type of care- conservative, interventional, palliative

Action: Prompt action saves lives. No vacillation

CT staging of the extent of the problem will help to define if the patient can be treated as an outpatient or inpatient. It defines patients who can be managed conservatively or with interventional radiology or surgery.

CT Staging Hinchey Classification

- Stage 0: Minimal diverticulitis with thickening of colon
- Stage 1: Peri colic inflammation or mesocolic abscess
- Stage 2: Distant or deep pelvic abscess with diverticulitis
- Stage 3: Purulent peritonitis with or without free gas and diverticulitis
- Stage 4: Faecal peritonitis—findings similar to stage 3

The complications of diverticulitis are as follows.

1. Diverticular bleeding
2. Diverticulitis
3. Obstruction
4. Perforation leading to localised or generalised peritonitis such as (4 P's):
   a. Pericolic abscess
   b. Paracolic abscess
   c. Pelvic abscess
   d. Peritonitis

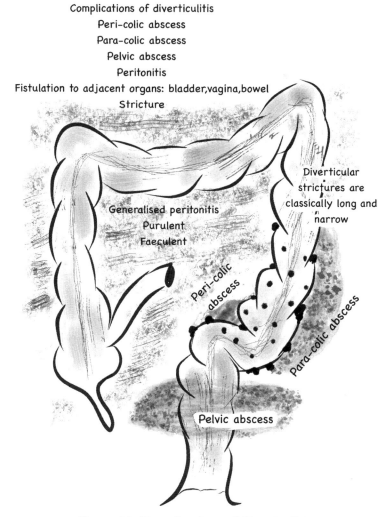

Complications of diverticulitis
Peri-colic abscess
Para-colic abscess
Pelvic abscess
Peritonitis
Fistulation to adjacent organs: bladder,vagina,bowel
Stricture

Diverticular strictures are classically long and narrow

Generalised peritonitis
Purulent
Faeculent

Peri-colic abscess

Para-colic abscess

Pelvic abscess

Figure 23: Complications of diverticulitis

When the perforation is contained locally, it manifests as an abscess around the colon. In the absence of containment, either due to the failure of the omentum and adjacent loops of bowel to isolate and wall off the collection or due to an overwhelmingly large perforation, it manifests as generalised peritonitis.

The management of the patient depends upon the severity of presentation. Patients with free perforation and peritonitis will be unstable and in a state of sepsis. The sepsis protocol must be implemented immediately. Early intervention saves lives.

Once stabilised and the results of the investigations are available, further treatment options will need consideration. As always these include several options. Many of these patients are elderly and are likely to have multiple comorbidities, including dementia. The decision to progress to surgery must be made after discussions with the patient (if able) and family or surrogates.

Treatment Options

- Feasibility of an operation is not an indication for its performance. Treatment is defined by careful assessment of every patient
- Non-interventional versus interventional options should be based on comorbidities and quality of life
- Wishes of the patient and family should be taken into consideration where the quality of life is poor
- Best interest meeting may be needed to decide on the management in the absence of capacity
- Non-operative management with antibiotics and monitoring will remain an option for some
- Non-operative management with radiologically placed drainage (i.e., interventional radiology) may need consideration in selected cases
- Surgical resection with or without primary anastomosis after resection may be an option for fit patients
- Always involve other specialities, especially critical care teams to define level of care peri-operatively
- End of life team will need to be consulted if that is the most appropriate decision for the patient

Surgical management could be laparoscopically assisted, open drainage, or resection. This will include primary anastomosis or end colostomy with a Hartmann's procedure.

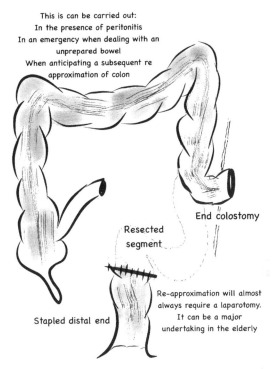

This is can be carried out:
In the presence of peritonitis
In an emergency when dealing with an
unprepared bowel
When anticipating a subsequent re
approximation of colon

End colostomy

Resected
segment

Re-approximation will almost
always require a laparotomy.
It can be a major
undertaking in the elderly

Stapled distal end

Figure 24: End colostomy—Hartmann's procedure

After resection, the proximal end can be brought out as an end colostomy. The distal end can be stapled and left within the pelvis, allowing for the possibility of re-approximation of the two ends at a later stage. The operation therefore becomes a two-stage procedure. All patients may not be suitable for this staged re-anastomosis because it will include further anaesthesia and surgery and may increase the morbidity if not the mortality. Some may be more willing and accepting of a permanent stoma.

Colostomy

Opening of the colon to the exterior is called a colostomy much as opening of the stomach is a gastrostomy, the ileum an ileostomy; jejunum a jejunostomy, and the caecum a caecostomy. The colon can be brought out in several ways.

Types of Colostomies

End colostomy is brought out of the abdominal wall. The distal segment is either stapled, as shown earlier, or it can be brought out of the abdomen when it is referred to as a mucous fistula.

In a defunctioning colostomy, the two ends are brought out side by side after complete resection of the intervening colon. This enables re approximation without the need for another laparotomy. It defunctions the distal bowel, and there is no possibility for ingress of faeces into the distal segment as the intervening bowel has been completely divided.

In a loop colostomy, a loop of bowel is exteriorised in continuity without division or resection. It may not technically defunction the distal segment as faeces can flow through to the distal segment since continuity is retained. The advantage of this procedure is the ease of carrying it out in an emergency and the relative ease of reversal.

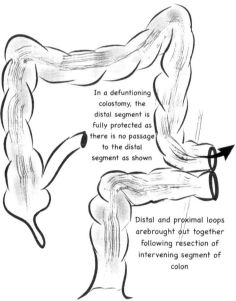

In a defuntioning colostomy, the distal segment is fully protected as there is no passage to the distal segment as shown

Distal and proximal loops arebrought out together following resection of intervening segment of colon

This type of colostomy, requires a satisfactory length of distal segment or enable it to be exteriorised.
It permits reversal without the need for a laparotomy as the ends can be mobilised, approximated and reduced without re-opening the abdomen with a formal laparotomy

Figure 25: Defunctioning colostomy

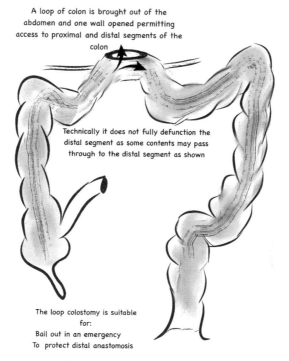

A loop of colon is brought out of the abdomen and one wall opened permitting access to proximal and distal segments of the colon

Technically it does not fully defunction the distal segment as some contents may pass through to the distal segment as shown

The loop colostomy is suitable for:
Bail out in an emergency
To protect distal anastomosis

Figure 26: Loop colostomy

In certain situations, the terminal ileum can be exteriorised, and once again it can be either an end ileostomy or a loop ileostomy.

Complications of all types of stomas include the following:

- Retraction due to muco-cutaneous separation
- Prolapse—protrusion due to peristaltic force
- Stenosis—due to narrowing
- Parastomal herniation
- Loss of blood supply causing ischaemia

Hartmann's Operation

Henri Albert Hartmann was a French surgeon who described this operation in 1921. In his time, before the days of antibiotics the mortality rate was high. Miles, in 1908 had developed the operation of abdomino-perineal resection for rectal cancer. That was a major undertaking and Hartman noted this procedure in his patients had a mortality rate of 38%. To reduce the mortality, Hartmann resected the tumour from the abdomen and closed the distal end. He brought out the proximal end as a colostomy. He presented the procedure in 34 patients, 3 of whom died; thus, his overall operative mortality was only 8.8%.

Hartmann never reversed the colostomy fearing that the mortality would be too high.

This paper is available online at http://www.grandrounds-e-med.com.

ANORECTAL PROBLEMS

Haemorrhoids commonly present with rectal bleeding. The presentation is very often one of painless and copious bleeding, causing anxiety.

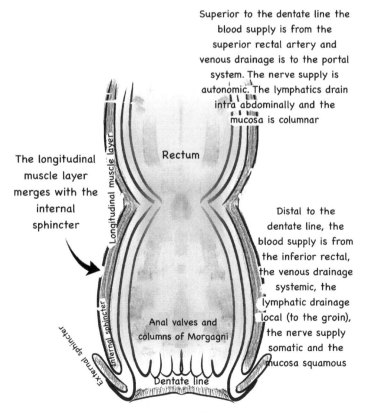

The lower four centimetres of the alimentary canal is very complex and controls the emptying process. Above all it differentiates flatus from faeces!

Superior to the dentate line the blood supply is from the superior rectal artery and venous drainage is to the portal system. The nerve supply is autonomic. The lymphatics drain intra abdominally and the mucosa is columnar

The longitudinal muscle layer merges with the internal sphincter

Longitudinal muscle layer

Rectum

Distal to the dentate line, the blood supply is from the inferior rectal, the venous drainage systemic, the lymphatic drainage local (to the groin), the nerve supply somatic and the mucosa squamous

External sphincter

Internal sphincter

Anal valves and columns of Morgagni

Dentate line

Figure 27: Anatomy of the anal canal

Haemorrhoids are mucosal cushions that are stretched over time and vascularised with enlarged veins.

Thicker calibre stools flatten mucosal folds preventing it from being stretched during voiding. Narrow calibre stools when voided stretch mucosal folds leading to mucosal cushion defects over time

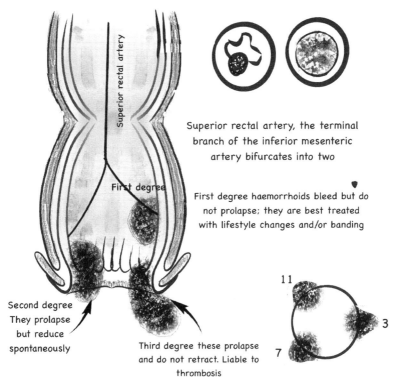

Superior rectal artery, the terminal branch of the inferior mesenteric artery bifurcates into two

First degree haemorrhoids bleed but do not prolapse; they are best treated with lifestyle changes and/or banding

Second degree
They prolapse but reduce spontaneously

Third degree these prolapse and do not retract. Liable to thrombosis

Haemorrhoids above the dentate line are called internal haemorrhoids. They are staged from 1 to 3 degrees. Haemorrhoids below dentate line are external haemorrhoids and seldom need intervention except for cosmesis

The Primary haemorrhoids are located at, 3, 7 and 11 O' clock positions. Secondary haemorrhoids are located in between the primary haemorrhoids

Figure 28: Anatomy of haemorrhoids

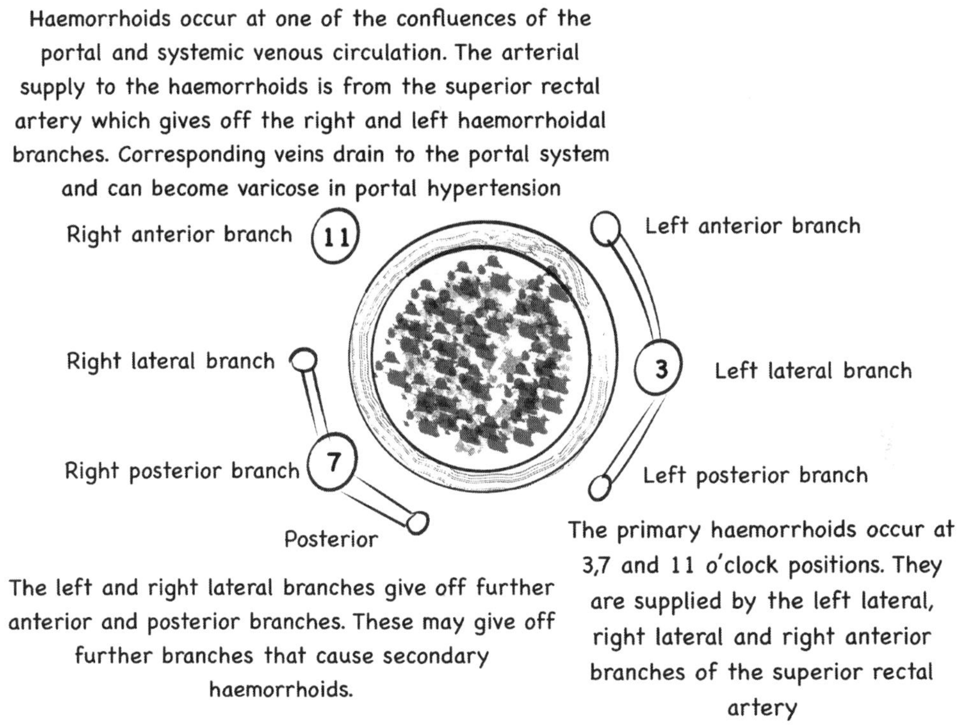

Haemorrhoids occur at one of the confluences of the portal and systemic venous circulation. The arterial supply to the haemorrhoids is from the superior rectal artery which gives off the right and left haemorrhoidal branches. Corresponding veins drain to the portal system and can become varicose in portal hypertension

Right anterior branch (11)   Left anterior branch

Right lateral branch ○   (3) Left lateral branch

Right posterior branch (7)   Left posterior branch

Posterior

The left and right lateral branches give off further anterior and posterior branches. These may give off further branches that cause secondary haemorrhoids.

The primary haemorrhoids occur at 3,7 and 11 o'clock positions. They are supplied by the left lateral, right lateral and right anterior branches of the superior rectal artery

Figure 29: Blood supply of haemorrhoids

Common Causes of Rectal Bleeding

- Haemorrhoids
- Fissure in ano
- Proctitis and inflammatory bowel disease
- Cancers and polyps of the colon and rectum
- Diverticular disease
- Trauma

> ## Rectal bleeding
>
> **Haemorrhoids**   Bright red Blood on the paper or in the pan
> Normally separate from the stools
> May be accompanied by a prolapsing mass that reduces spontaneously
> or with manual assistance
> **Neoplasia**   Dark blood with or without mucous; bright if the tumour
> is low in the rectum. Blood is normally mixed with stools
> **Inflammatory Bowel Disease** Bright blood, mucous and loose stools
> **These signs overlap and there is a wide grey zone**

Haemorrhoids are defined as mucosal cushion defects in which the vessels become prominent and present like varicosities of the veins. Haemorrhoidal bleeding is normally painless and often tends to be noted on paper or in the pan.

Haemorrhoids usually occur at 3,7 and 11'O-Clock positions due to the distribution of the superior rectal vessels. The pathophysiology is varied but it is related to the erect human posture and longstanding straining at stools. When the stools are of a thick calibre, the mucosal folds of the rectum get compressed against the wall and the folds are flattened. On the other hand, the mucosal folds are prominent when the calibre of the stools is narrow or if the stools are pellety. On voiding, the mucosal folds are stretched as the stools are extruded. This recurrent process of stretching and relaxing over long periods, tends to make the mucosa lax leading to mucosal cushion defects. In time, the mucosal cushions are stretched and filled with blood vessels. The precipitating cause may be episodes of constipation; however, this is not exclusively the case. In some it follows a period of loose stools. Pregnancy with related increase in pelvic pressure can also lead to haemorrhoids. In patients with portal hypertension the ano- rectal veins are areas of porta-systemic anastamosis with the dentate line being the watershed between the two systems; above it the drainage is to the portal system and below it to the systemic veins. The anorectum at the level of the dentate line is an area where there is anastomosis between the systemic and portal systems. The superior rectal veins drain to the portal vein and these do not have valves. The hydrostatic pressure is therefore transmitted vertically from the portal vein and there is communication with the inferior rectal veins that drain into the Venacava. This leads to varicosities of the veins presenting as haemorrhoids.

Precipitating Factors

- Constipation
- Loose stools
- Pregnancy
- Portal hypertension
- Posture
- Patients on anticoagulants

The key points to note regarding rectal bleeding are as follows.

- Haemorrhoidal bleeding is normally bright red and painless.
- Painful bleeding is often associated with fissure in ano.
- In haemorrhoidal bleeding, the stools are separate from the blood.
- Constipation is a precursor in many cases of fissure and haemorrhoids, but not always.
- Blood is noted on paper on wiping or on the pan.
- Blood in the pan appears to be a lot more due to dilution and is commonly haemorrhoidal.
- Blood on the paper could be due to fissure as well as haemorrhoids.
- Mucous and blood is common with inflammatory disease.
- Diverticular bleed can be profuse.

Management of Rectal Bleeding

As always, a good history is important in elucidating the cause of the presentation. Lifestyle changes will need discussions with the patient, including avoidance of constipation and not sitting on the 'loo for more than a minute and two'.

A digital rectal examination is mandatory. This may not be possible in patients with fissure in ano as the acute condition is very painful. The fissure may be visible on inspection, often being located just at the anal verge at the six or twelve o'clock positions. However, where there is doubt, an examination under anaesthesia is needed to exclude other causes such as a painful thrombosed piles or malignancy. A sigmoidoscopy is needed to confirm the diagnosis and exclude other causes.

Polyps or cancers of the rectum can present as haemorrhoids.

Colonoscopy may be needed if the cause of the rectal bleeding is not obvious. This is likely to be the case when the patient is older and offers a family history of bowel cancer. It may also be indicated when the type of bleeding is thought not to be related to anorectal pathology based on the history.

Faecal calprotectin is a marker of inflammation of the bowel. This may be needed in patients who present with rectal bleeding associated with change in bowel habit.

Proctoscopy and a digital rectal examination is needed in all patients presenting with a clear history of bright red rectal bleeding that is separate from stools; this alone is likely to define the cause. Proctoscopy will help locate the site of the haemorrhoids and assist in planning further treatment.

Fissure in ano may cause rectal bleeding similar to haemorrhoids with the distinction that fissures are painful.

Typically, painful rectal bleeding where the pain lasts for a few hours after voiding is consistent with a fissure rather than haemorrhoids, although thrombosed haemorrhoids or a perianal haematoma can present likewise. In patients with a fissure in ano, the patient will volunteer the information that voiding stools is like passing glass.

Perianal haematoma, however, presents with acute pain that is followed by a lump in the perineum. The lump is due to bleed into an external skin tag or into the skin. It swells and becomes painful due to the pressure that builds in the contained space. Release of tension by opening the haematoma resolves the pain. On the other hand, if a nonoperative approach is followed, the relief occurs with resorption of the haematoma that normally takes place in about five days; this is thus referred to as the 'five day painful condition'.

Management of Haemorrhoids

First degree

- Dietary changes to avoid constipation.
- Laxatives to reduce straining at stools.
- Reassurance that it is self-limiting in most.
- Banding of haemorrhoids if persistent. This involves placing a tight rubber band on the base of the haemorrhoids above the dentate line to prevent pain. Over a few days, the haemorrhoid denuded of blood supply falls away.

Second degree

- Banding of haemorrhoids along with the treatment for first degree.
- Haemorrhoidal artery ligation operation, where the feeding vessels are identified by ultrasound and ligated under anaesthesia, is another less invasive procedure when the bleeding is persistent. The success rate is variably predicted at 70 per cent.

Third degree

These will require a traditional haemorrhoidectomy (Milligan and Morgan). The internal sphincter is identified and kept out of harm's way. The haemorrhoids are then excised and the wound can be left open or closed depending on the type of operation favoured. The procedure is painful post-operatively, and first bowel movement after operation can be very painful.

Skin bridges must be maintained between excisions to ensure that fibrosis does not result in an anal stenosis. Increasingly these are less commonly done, with early intervention being the norm.

Classically, the primary haemorrhoids are located at the three, seven, and eleven o'clock positions. The secondary haemorrhoids are located in between the primary haemorrhoids. When there are multiple haemorrhoids, the adage, 'If it is a clover, the story is over, but if it is a dahlia, it is a sure failure.' is likely to be true. Secondary haemorrhoids can be difficult to treat.

Denis Parsons Burkitt a young British surgeon whilst working in Africa drew attention to the importance of bulk in preventing colorectal problems. He collected data on the weight and bulk of the stools of the people in Southern Africa. He noted that when the stool weight was high the ano rectal and colon problems were low. He supposedly influenced Kellogg cereal company about the benefit of fibre. The founder Kellog was himself a doctor. Fibre the indigestible part of plants, was added to Kelloggs' breakfast cereals. The fibre removed in processing was replaced in the cereals to aid in bulking the stools. It isn't entirely clear that this approach to bulking the stools confers similar benefits to that provided by nature! The current recommendation is that more helpings of vegetables and fruit will provide the protective bulk. One helping is one handful. There is a debate as to how many handfuls are needed, but the take home message is clear. Diet is destiny! Burkitt is famously quoted as saying " if you have small stools, you need to build big hospitals"!

Thrombosed Haemorrhoids

Occasionally, when a patient has third-degree haemorrhoids, the vessels in the prolapsed haemorrhoids may get occluded. This can lead to painful thrombosis.

Presentation is acute with a perianal lump that is very painful and tender. There is unlikely to be any bleeding, and pain will be the most common presentation, along with a persistent prolapse.

Management with rest, elevation, and cold packs may relieve the pain and temporise the situation, allowing for an elective haemorrhoidectomy at a later date. In some patients, the symptoms fail to resolve, and they benefit from immediate surgery. In the days prior to the advent of antibiotics, this was a dreaded operation leading to complications of portal pyaemia and sepsis. It is necessary, therefore, to provide patients with appropriate antibiotic cover prior to emergency haemorrhoidectomy.

Perianal Haematoma

As stated earlier, it is referred to as the 'five-day painful lump' because its settles down spontaneously in most, leaving just a skin tag. If the pain is very severe, bisecting the lump and evacuating the thrombus relieves the pain instantly.

Perianal Crohn's

This is a very difficult condition to treat surgically. In most cases, there will be a history of Crohn's. In the perineum, there is likely to be thickened fleshy tags with persistent discomfort. Surgery is not indicated, but a biopsy may be needed in some to confirm the histology and initiate medical management.

Fissure in Ano

A fissure in ano is a tear in the anal mucosa exposing the internal sphincter. The presentation may be acute with severe pain on defaecation; there may be associated blood on the paper but seldom if ever in the pan. On examination, the tear is seen on inspection at the anal verge on just spreading the buttocks. When the problem is chronic, there may be a skin tag extending from the lower limit of the fissure, which is referred to as a sentinel tag. In general, the tear is common posteriorly at about the six o'clock position in most, however in women, anterior tears at twelve o'clock occur in about 40 per cent of patients. The pathophysiology is thought to be stretching at voiding stools, leading an area of ischaemia, which then gives way leading to a fissure. It can also occur during childbirth and after anal intercourse. Ageing may also be a factor, although constipation is more likely to be the cause of the tear.

Management of Fissure in Ano

The principle here is to relieve pain mostly by reducing the spasm that follows voiding. This is done by:

- Softening the stools
- Application of local anaesthetic such as lidocaine 5%
- Relieving smooth muscle spasm with agents such as Rectogesic (GTN) or Diltiazem
- Injecting Botox if the above treatment options fail. This is given in small quantities in the intersphincteric plane.
- Temporary loss of continence, especially for flatus, will need addressing during consent
- Lateral sphincterotomy is the gold standard. The sphincter is divided at about the three o'clock position away from the six o'clock position, the common location of the fissure.
- In women, especially those who have had children, it is best to assess the status of the sphincter with an ultra sound examination prior to surgery; there is an increased risk of problems with continence.

Fistula in ano

These are not uncommon problems.
The presentation can be with:

- Faecal soiling
- Perianal discomfort
- Perianal abscess

Low fistulae can be laid open with minimal risk to continence. Techniques to block the channel with glue or excising it fully have met with variable success. All patients need careful assessment and discussion prior to surgery. The key principle is to avoid breaching the sphincter and causing more harm.

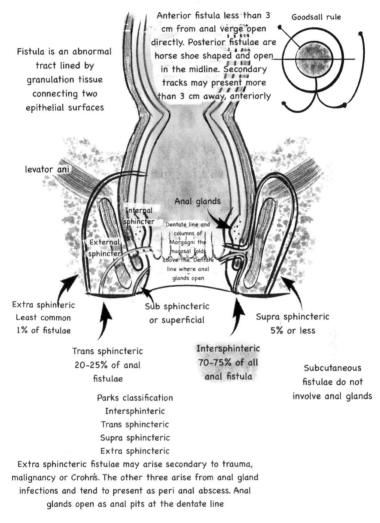

Figure 30: Fistula in ano

Problems with Anal Continence

This is an area where specialist expertise is needed. The problem is not uncommon in the elderly and very often affects women. Many patients present in their seventh and eighth decades.

The loss of continence can arise in the following:

- Women who have had protracted and prolonged labour in years past
- Patients with neurological problems
- Patients who have had perianal trauma
- Those rare patients who have had complications of surgery such as sphincterotomy and haemorrhoidectomy
- Those who have laxity of neuromuscular mechanisms

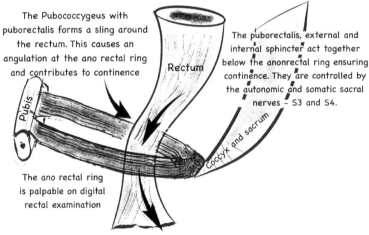

The Pubococcygeus with puborectalis forms a sling around the rectum. This causes an angulation at the ano rectal ring and contributes to continence

The puborectalis, external and internal sphincter act together below the anorectal ring ensuring continence. They are controlled by the autonomic and somatic sacral nerves – S3 and S4.

The ano rectal ring is palpable on digital rectal examination

Eisenhammer noted that the ring of white fibres surrounding the anal canal at its lower end is the INTERNAL and not the external sphincter; under anaesthesia or on pushing the internal sphincter lies internal but lower than the external sphincter

Anal resting tone on manometry, 2 cm proximal to the anal verge is around 50-60mmHg. It is higher in men than women

Morgan and Thompson noted that the internal and external sphincters function like two telescoped tubes. The muscle in the floor of fissures is the internal sphincter. Goligher stated that division of the internal sphincter at sphinterotomy carries a 30% risk of faecal soiling

Figure 31 Mechanisms of anal continence

ABDOMINAL TRAUMA

Abdominal trauma is of two types: blunt injury and penetrating injury. Blunt injury is common after road traffic accidents. Penetrating injury is fortunately less common and follows stabs and gunshot injuries, accounting for less than one-fourth of abdominal injuries.

Trauma teams are now set up across all hospitals in the UK, but it is important to know the principles of management. When confronted with major abdominal trauma, the damage is done due to bleeding and hypothermia, leading to the 'lethal triad'.

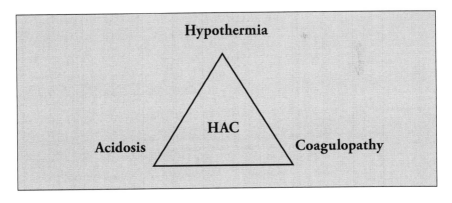

The mortality rises exponentially as the lethal triad sets in, and it is thus important to prevent it where possible by controlling blood loss and hypothermia. When uncontrolled, coagulation cascade is affected, leading to more bleeding. This was recognised in the 1980s during operations for trauma (Stone 1983).

The term 'damage control surgery' was coined by Rotondo and Schwab (1993) to describe a three-stage management of patients with major abdominal trauma.

Damage Control Surgery

Phase 1:   Control of bleeding

Control of contamination

Closure – temporary

Phase 2:   Restoration of physiology in ITU

Phase 3:   Re Operation

Restoration of anatomy

Re-establishment of bowel continuity

Following a rapid initial surgery—abbreviated laparotomy—the abdomen may or may not be closed. Bleeding sites are controlled with ligation, packing (pack and pause), or splenectomy when needed. Bowel ends are exteriorised after lavage.

The abdomen is not closed fully to avoid intra-abdominal hypertension. In the 1980s, it was noted that sustained intra-abdominal hypertension rapidly led to renal dysfunction. By leaving the abdomen open, the physiology is restored. In certain situations, a colectomy leaving both the stapled ends within the abdomen followed by return to theatre in twenty-four to forty-eight hours will obviate the need for colostomy. Re-establishment of intestinal continuity can be achieved without the need for a stoma.

> **World Society of Abdominal Compartment Syndrome Guidelines 2013**
>
> **IAH** – intra abdominal hypertension is defined as a sustained pathological elevation of intra-abdominal pressure ≥12mmHg
>
> | Grade I | IAP 12-15 mmHg |
> | Grade II | IAP 16-20 mmHg |
> | Grade III | IAP 21-25 mmHg |
> | Grade IV | IAP > 25 mmHg |

When massive blood transfusion is needed (defined as greater than ten units in twenty-four hours, or three units in one hour), it is important to involve the haematology team at the outset to ensure that the complex coagulation process can be supported from the outset and not be allowed to be consumed, leading to consumption coagulopathy. This requires not only volume by way of fluids but also coagulation factors, platelets, and RBCs to transport oxygen in the presence of ongoing haemorrhagic shock.

> **Massive Transfusion Protocol - MTP**
>
> 1. Haemorrhage is the most cause of death in the first 24 hours after trauma
> 2. Plasma – Platelet – RBC ratio of 1:1:1 reduces exsanguination
> 3. Cryoprecipitate and Tranexamic Acid (1gm in 10 mins) may need to be considered
> 4. Delay in reaching targets increases mortality
> 5. Reaching targets in 6 hours saves more lives
> 6. 'Going big early' decreases the need for more blood products and is beneficial in the overall management (based on UK trauma protocol manual)

Criteria for initiating Massive Transfusion Protocol

1. Systolic blood pressure <90 mmhg
2. Heart rate <120/min
3. pH 7.24 or less
4. Focused scan for trauma (FAST) positive

In haemorrhagic shock, there is an inability of the physiological system to meet the needs of the oxygen demand of the organs. As a ready rule of thumb, 200 mL of packed red cells will increase the haematocrit by three in the absence of continued bleeding.

Stages of Haemorrhagic Shock in a 70 Kg Adult

Parameter	Class 1	Class 2	Class 3	Class 4
Blood loss (mL)	< 750	750–1500	1500–2000	> 2000
Blood loss (%)	< 15	15–30	30–40	> 40
Heart rate	< 100	> 100	> 120	> 140
Blood pressure	Normal	Orthostatic hypotension	Hypotensive	Severely hypotensive
Mentation	Normal	Mildly Anxious	Confused	Confused withdrawn

The principles of management are the same as outlined previously, but senior staff from multiple specialities will need to be involved from the outset.

GYNAECOLOGICAL EMERGENCIES

Gynaecological emergencies relate to pelvic inflammatory disease and ectopic pregnancy, which may masquerade as lower abdominal or right iliac fossa pain. These patients may present directly to the surgeons. It is worth reiterating that in all young women, the routine protocol to follow must always include urine for nitrates and beta HCG.

If nitrite is positive, then a mid-stream urine sample must be sent for culture and sensitivity prior to initiating antibiotic therapy as per the hospital's protocol.

If the beta HCG is positive in the presence of abdominal pain, then the gynaecological team must be informed about the patient.

If there is suspicion of pelvic pathology a pelvic ultrasound examination must be arranged urgently; this is mandatory if the beta HCG is positive because ectopic pregnancy must be excluded.

In certain situations, it may not be clear if there is a pelvic pathology such as a tubo-ovarin mass or an appendicular pathology. It is best to work in conjunction with the gynaecologists, and at times a combined laparoscopy may be needed.

UROLOGICAL EMERGENCIES

The common urological problems that present to acute surgery are as follows:

1. Renal colic
2. Haematuria
3. Retention of urine
4. Torsion of testis
5. Epididymo-orchitis

Renal colic occurs due to the progressive movement of kidney stones along the ureter.

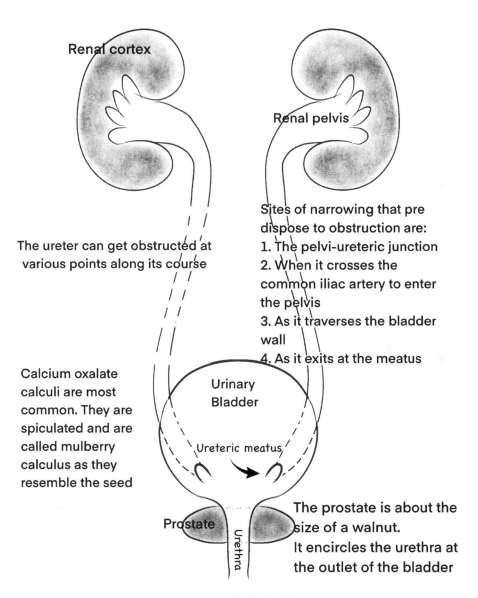

Renal cortex

Renal pelvis

The ureter can get obstructed at various points along its course

Sites of narrowing that pre dispose to obstruction are:
1. The pelvi-ureteric junction
2. When it crosses the common iliac artery to enter the pelvis
3. As it traverses the bladder wall
4. As it exits at the meatus

Calcium oxalate calculi are most common. They are spiculated and are called mulberry calculus as they resemble the seed

Urinary Bladder

Ureteric meatus

Prostate

Urethra

The prostate is about the size of a walnut.
It encircles the urethra at the outlet of the bladder

Figure 32: Sites of calculi obstruction

The common stones are as follows:

- **Calcium oxalate stones**—Most common, small, and spiculated like a mulberry seed. Spicules can cause microscopic haematuria as they move down the ureter. It is not associated with urinary infection, and the urine is more likely to be acidic. This type of stone presents classically with colic from loin to groin. With each episode of colic, the stone moves down the ureter.
- **Triple phosphate stones**—These may not cause symptoms and can occur silently. They can lead to bilateral obstruction and renal failure. They can occur during pregnancy as there may be urinary stasis. They are very often associated with urinary infection. The urine is likely to be alkaline. Normally they progress slowly and occupy the entire renal pelvis and calyces, appearing like the horn of a stag—hence called the stag horn calculus.
- Urate stones, Cystine xanthine stones are less common and occur due to metabolic problems.

The principles of management relate to pain relief followed by diagnosis and referral to the urologists. NSAIDS are the drug of choice (NICE guidance). If NSAIDS are contraindicated, then intravenous paracetamol or opioids can be prescribed. It is worth noting that 90 per cent of renal stones are detectable on plain X-rays as opposed to gallstones where 90 per cent are invisible on plain X-rays.

Examination of the urine for nitrates and blood is mandatory. If ureteric colic is suspected, a low-dose, non-contrast CT urogram must be arranged urgently. If this is delayed, the opportunity to make the diagnosis may be lost if the stone passes.

Treatment depends on size and site of the stone.

- Wait and watch policy is acceptable for stones smaller than 5 mm
- Medical expulsive therapy can be tried with alpha blocker for lower ureteric stones smaller than 10 mm
- Extra corporeal Shockwave lithotripsy (ESWL) can be used for larger stones. This breaks the stones and allows for natural passage

- Percutaneous nephrolithotomy (PCNL), is a procedure that is used when the stone is in the kidney or upper ureter and is too large to be broken by other techniques. It is carried out with a tiny incision in the flank with percutaneous cannulation of the kidney and ureter under radiological guidance. The stone is extracted through this procedure or broken down with a lithotripter and extracted in pieces.
- Surgical extraction

Serum calcium levels must be assessed to exclude hyper parathyroid disorders.

The urinary calcium must be estimated in all with recurring colic. They may be voiding more calcium in the urine (hypercalciuria) and may benefit from diuretic therapy.

Prevention of recurrence may be assisted by advising the consumption of more water. Whilst it is nice to advise two or three litres of fluids a day, it may not always be practical as patients vary in weight. Asking a patient to drink enough to ensure that the colour of the water that is passed nearly approximates the colour of the water that is drunk works well in principle. It ensures that the urine passed is dilute.

Haematuria

The presence of blood in the urine can be non-visible or visible.

Nonvisible haematuria (NVH) can be due to urinary tract infections, benign prostatic hypertrophy, and ureteric colic. This is also referred to a microscopic haematuria.

Visible or macroscopic haematuria are mostly due to urological tumours such as bladder polyps and malignancies in the kidney, ureter, bladder or prostate.

Management is through the haematuria clinic or the two-week wait pathway under the urologists.

Urinary Retention

Common causes:

- Prostatic enlargement
- Post-operative
- Urethral stricture
- Drugs

Urinary retention can be acute or chronic. Acute retention is a common problem and can be due to prostatic enlargement, leading to obstruction of the urethra. It can also occur following surgery under regional anaesthesia such as spinal or even after general anaesthesia. It can follow from drugs such as tricyclic antidepressants and sympathomimetics. These can affect the function of the detrusor muscle of the bladder. Urethral strictures can also cause outflow obstruction.

Prostatism

Commonly, patients with prostatic hypertrophy will have symptoms of outflow obstruction sometimes leading to acute retention of urine in the bladder. The symptoms include nocturia, hesitancy, and precipitancy for a considerable time prior to an acute presentation with retention of urine. Whilst acute retention is painful, many patients with chronic retention may have a very distended bladder without any symptoms.

The treatment is by catheterisation and referral to a urology service. Once catheterised, a trial without catheter can be initiated after treatment for forty-eight hours with an alpha-adrenergic blocker such as Tamsulosin. Once again urinary cultures are needed to ensure early and appropriate treatment of infections. The cause of the prostatic enlargement will need to be ascertained.

Epididymo-orchitis and testicular torsions present with testicular pain. The diagnosis of torsion may be confirmed with a Doppler ultrasound examination. Current recommendation, however, is to proceed to surgery on suspicion of torsion of the testis. If Doppler studies are done and if they are ambivalent, then an exploration under anaesthesia is mandatory to exclude torsion of the testis.

In infants, infantile scrotal oedema, a condition where there is oedema of the scrotum with normal testes can present acutely with a swelling causing anxiety to parents. An ultrasound is needed to reassure the parents that there is no torsion.

Epididymo-orchitis is inflammation of the testis and epididymis
Onset is likely to be gradual and may be associated with urinary infection, (mostly bacterial) in the older age group
It must be distinguished from torsion which presents acutely in the younger age group

Intra vaginal torsion occurs when a testis with a horizontal lie and a mesorchium undergoes torsion within the tunica vaginalis
The horizontal lie of the testis - 'clapper in a bell position' can be recognised clinically when not acute

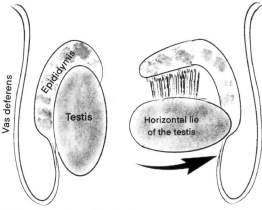

In all patients presenting with acute testicular pain when torsion is suspected surgical intervention is preferable to a Doppler study. All investigations have a false negative rate and it is preferable to explore surgically immediately than wait for investigations

Intravaginal torsion may present with right iliac fossa pain mimicking sppendicitis

Extravaginal torsion involving the testis and epididymis is more common in infants with an undescended testis
This may present as a tender groin lump and an empty scrotum in an infant

Testis has a tiny 'appendix' - the hydatid of Morgagni, which may also undergo torsion. Where the testis is non tender and the presentation is one of acute testicular pain an immediate Doppler study may show a normal blood supply to the testis
Infantile scrotal oedema is a condition where the testis is non tender but there is scrotal oedema

Figure 33: Torsion testis and epididymis

VASCULAR EMERGENCIES

The abdominal aorta bifurcates just below and to the left of the umbilicus to form the common iliac vessels. These in turn bifurcate into external and internal iliac arteries. The external iliac artery continues as the common femoral artery that bifurcates into the superficial and profounda femoral arteries

At sites of bifurcation there is turbulence. Turbulence damages the intima and initiates plaque formation

These main large vessels are the vessels of conductance
They are affected by atherosclerotic process
The distal tertiary smaller branches are the vessels of supply that are affected by diabetes

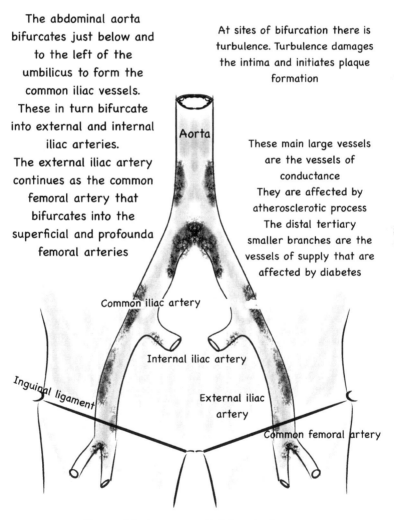

Aorta

Common iliac artery

Internal iliac artery

Inguinal ligament

External iliac artery

Common femoral artery

Figure 34: Anatomy of abdominal aorta

The abdominal aorta bifurcates into the common iliac arteries just below and to the left of the umbilicus. For surface marking, obesity must be taken into consideration, but even so this site is a reliable location for bifurcation, as noted in CT studies of the abdomen.

The Common iliac artery bifurcates into internal and external iliac arteries; external iliac artery continues as the common femoral artery and this bifurcates deep to the inguinal ligament to the superficial femoral and deep femoral (profunda femoris) arteries. The superficial femoral artery continues as the popliteal artery and bifurcates into the anterior and posterior tibial arteries, with the posterior tibial giving off the peroneal artery. There is thus a common pattern of bifurcation down the aorta.

Vessels of conductance are the main vessels that conduct blood to the body from the heart. These bifurcate all along the limbs. At points of bifurcation, turbulence affects streamline flow and causes intimal damage, which becomes the focus of atherosclerosis. The process, therefore affects the large vessels.

Vessels of supply are the small vessels that take blood to the muscles branching off from conductance vessels. They are typically affected by diabetes.

Lipid retention in the wall of the vessels leads to chronic inflammation at the sites where there is turbulence. The process starts very early in childhood as fatty streaks. These progress to fibrous plaques that are capable of rupturing. Progression with sub intimal deposition of lipid over time leads to stenosis and thrombosis. The entire process proceeds variably in people, facilitated by genetic susceptibility in some with hyperlipidaemic states and worsened in some by hypertension, diabetes, smoking, obesity, ageing, and as always diet. Diet is destiny!

Atherosclerotic disease predominantly affects the vessels of conductance, the proximal vessels. The presentation can be acute or chronic, the latter being more common.

Predisposing Factors

- Smoking
- Obesity
- Hypertension
- Diabetes
- Hyperlipidaemia

Patients with chronic limb ischaemia are invariably smokers or ex-smokers, and a history of smoking must always be obtained.

Chronic Critical lower limb ischaemia

- **Persistent pain** in the foot for more than 48 hrs despite opiate analgesia
- Presence of **tissue necrosis or gangrene**
- **Absolute Doppler pressure** of less than 50mmhg in a non-diabetic or 30mmhg in a diabetic

---

Progressive intermittent claudication is an important symptom, and this history must be elicited. Claudication is pain precipitated by activity such as walking, and Fontaine is credited with the staging.

Stage I— 'Walk through' calf pain. The pain in the calf resolves on walking as more and **more collateral vessels are recruited to deliver more oxygen** to the peripheral tissues and wash away the metabolites of anaerobic respiration. The pain is in the muscles of activity, the calf in the lower limbs.

Stage II—Rest relieves calf pain. The recruitment of collateral vessels is insufficient to deliver the needed oxygen to the tissues. The muscular activity must therefore come to a stop to allow the tissues to rest and regain aerobic respiration.

Stage III—Foot pain at rest. The pain is in the distal most part, the foot. The oxygenation even at rest is inadequate to supply the peripheral requirements. The foot which is farthest from heart is unable to receive enough oxygen for its metabolic needs. This manifests as constant and severe pain.

Acute Thrombosis and Acute Embolism

This distinction is easy to explain, but it may sometimes be difficult to judge clinically. The management of the two tend to be different, and hence it is a crucial decision to make clinically albeit assisted by investigations. This will enable delivery of appropriate care.

When acute limb ischaemia is suspected, the vascular specialists must be informed and involved in further care. Suffice it to know that with acute embolism, the presentation is classical and the onset sudden. Many patients will have abnormal cardiac rhythms, with the commonest being atrial fibrillation. Thrombotic episode is more gradual, with a history of claudication and rest pain.

Acute limb ischaemia
Embolism
Thrombus
Trauma

Presentation – 5 P's
Pain or paraesthesia
Pallor
Pulselessness
Perishing cold
Paralysis

Embolism is associated with changes in cardiac rhythm, and in any acute presentation, atrial fibrillation or frequent ectopic beats may be present and must be looked for actively.

Investigations in vascular surgery are guided by a balance of principles that determine if the patient is safe for surgery and if the surgery is safe for the patient.

Ensure that the patient is safe for surgery.
Check all cardiovascular risk factors. 'Head over heart over heels' is the oft repeated statement that reiterates the fact that cerebral and **cardiac** systems must be examined and assessed along with the limbs. Most patients are arteriopaths with the process of atherosclerosis extending to all vessels in the body. Many will have comorbidities such as previous TIA, CVA, myocardial disease, hypertension and diabetes.

Ensure that surgery is safe for the patient.
There is little point in carrying out a major operation when a lesser procedure will suffice, such as an angioplasty as opposed to a major bypass. Safe surgery always depends on choosing the right patient for the right procedure.

A map of the vascular tree by way of an angiogram, MR angiogram, or duplex scanning is almost always needed. An ECG and coagulation studies are routine investigations in all patients presenting with vascular symptoms.

If there is critical limb ischaemia, consider one of two options.

- Limb-saving vascular reconstructive procedure
- Life-saving amputation, which may be below or above knee

Gangrene

Gangrene is defined as macroscopic death of tissue with putrefaction.

The key distinction is that gangrene is macroscopic as opposed to necrosis, which is microscopic death of tissue.

Gangrene occurs at the distal extremities when there is loss of blood supply. This can occur due to the following:

- Peripheral vascular disease
- Raynaud's disease
- Vasculitis
- Diabetes

Typically, gangrene can be wet or dry.

Gangrene

Dry Gangrene
- Seen in patients with **atherosclerotic** peripheral vascular disease
- Has a **well-defined line of demarcation**
- This line of demarcation is **Aseptic**

Wet Gangrene:
- Seen in **diabetic patients**
- Has an **ill-defined line of separation**
- This line of separation is **Infected**

Dry gangrene is associated with peripheral vascular disease. These patients present with constant foot pain if the vessels of the lower limb are affected. They may have a low-grade pyrexia. There is no infection, and the treatment will be directed towards the management of the associated limb ischaemia followed by an amputation of the gangrenous toe or part of the limb.

Wet gangrene is generally infected and occurs in the distal aspect of the foot in diabetic patients. These patients may benefit from antibiotic therapy, but eventually most will need an amputation. In many patients there is sensory loss, and the cause of the gangrene may be a trauma to the diabetic foot, leading to infection in the presence of a decreased blood supply.

Aneurysm of the Abdominal Aorta

Abdominal aortic aneurysm

Risk factors:
Smoking
Ageing
Male
White
Positive family history

The diameter of the infra renal aorta is 1.5 to 2 cm
The aorta is diagnosed as being aneurysmal when it
reaches a diameter of 3 cm or twice the diameter of
the proximal aorta

The operation may be:
Elective or an emergency
Open or endoscopic
Repaired with a
Straight or a trouser graft
(if common iliacs are
aneurysmal)

EVAR involves the
placement of a straight
or trouser graft in the
infra renal aorta through
the common femoral
artery under
radiological guidance
The absence of a long
midline incision makes
it less invasive and
useful in selected
patients with straight
iliac arteries which
facilitate placement of
graft

Risk of rupture
increases with
increasing diameter. At
a diameter of 5.5 cm
the risk benefit ratio
favours intervention in
an otherwise fit patient

Open operations carry a
greater risk in terms of
morbidity and mortality.
Endovascular aneurysm
repair(EVAR) has less
morbidity and mortality but
long term results favour
open procedures in
suitable patients

Open operations require
cross clamping of the aorta
increasing the after load and
strain on an already strained
heart bearing in mind most of
these patients are
arteriopathic

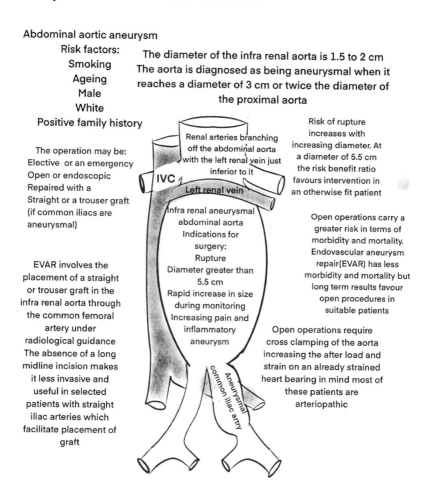

Renal arteries branching
off the abdominal aorta
with the left renal vein just
inferior to it

IVC

Left renal vein

Infra renal aneurysmal
abdominal aorta
Indications for
surgery:
Rupture
Diameter greater than
5.5 cm
Rapid increase in size
during monitoring
Increasing pain and
inflammatory
aneurysm

Aneurysmal
common iliac artry

On declamping after placement of the graft hypotension
can occur in the absence of effective pre loading prior
to declamping. This is due to vasodilatation on
reperfusion and can lead to acute kidney injury

Figure 35: Abdominal aortic aneurysm key points

ABSCESSES, BOILS, AND CARBUNCLES

No surgical discussion can overlook the common presentations that are confronted daily by surgeons. Abscesses can occur anywhere in the body but are common in areas subject to friction such as axilla, groin, perineum, and natal clefts.

Classically, abscess is defined as a cavity containing pus lined by granulation tissue and surrounded by cellulitis.

Boils or furuncles are infections of the root of hair follicles. When multiple boils occur in close approximation, it is referred to as a carbuncle. It involves the subcutaneous tissue and is accompanied by sloughing. These occur in the nape of the neck and back and are associated with diabetes.

> ## Coagulase positive staphylococcus aureus
>
> Cause **skin infections – ABC** – abscesses, boils and carbuncles
> **Coagulase** production by the staphylococcus helps it break down
> fibrinogen to fibrin on encountering blood. This coats the bacteria
> and prevents its recognition and phagocytosis.
>
> **Aureus** – Latin for gold, because of the golden yellow colonies
> surrounded by beta haemolysis it produces on **blood agar plates.**
>
> **Beta haemolysis** – is the breakdown of RBC by haemolysin produced
> by the bacteria. Many bacteria produce haemolysin, particularly
> staphylococcus and streptococcus

When the hair follicles get inflamed due to shaving or friction, they
infect the sweat glands in the skin and are referred to as hidradenitis. If it
suppurates, the condition is referred to as hidradenitis suppurativa. Once
again these occur in the axilla, groin, or perineum.

> ## MRSA – Methicillin resistant staphylococcus aureus
>
> Methicillin is a type of penicillin and bacteria that are resistant to it are
> also resistant to many commonly used antibiotics making it difficult
> to treat them.
>
> **Colonization or staphylococcal carriage** must be suspected when
> patients present with recurrent and multiple infections.
>
> **Decolonization** should be considered only when there is no infection
> and it involves clearing nasal and cutaneous carriage by application of
> **Hibiscrub** for skin and **Naseptin** (Hibiscrub and Neomycin) for nose.

Pilonidal abscess occurs commonly in the natal cleft of the perineum.
These occur due to infection of a pilonidal sinus. Pilonidal sinus is the
presence of sinus in the skin due to friction and maceration in moist

parts of the body such as the natal cleft and perineum. Pilar means hair and nidus, nest. It is a nest of hair at the base of a sinus. Typically it is formed of hair that has entered this 'nest' from exterior, noted by the fact that the roots of the hair are superficial with the ends being located deep. This indicates that the hair is a 'migrant' and not a local! Mostly hair that falls from the neck, collects in the natal cleft area. It was noted to be very common amongst American soldiers in the Korean War in the 1950's and came to be called the 'Jeep bottom'.

Perianal abscess can be secondary to a fistula in ano, or it can arise from the perianal skin. When associated with a fistula, the type of organism confronted is likely to be those that are commonly present in the bowel and not the skin. If the cultures grow E. Coli, Klebsiella, or Bacteroides then a fistula should be suspected. These will recur unless the underlying pathology is addressed. If, in contrast, staphylococcus is grown, it is more likely to be a cutaneous problem.

Hilton's Method of Incision and Drainage of an Abscess

All large abscesses need surgical drainage in the presence of fluctuation. In the perineum, it is best not to wait for fluctuation, and the abscess must be drained when the patient presents with acute perianal pain, preferably after localisation by aspiration under anaesthesia followed by incision and drainage. In areas where there are underlying nerves and vessels, the skin over the abscess is incised superficially in the direction of the underlying structures; the deep fascia is then punctured with a 'sinus forceps' that has a blunt tip, the cavity is entered, and locules are broken down. The wound is left open and packed lightly.

Role of Antibiotics

Antibiotic treatment is not needed for abscesses that are incised and drained, however they may be needed in some circumstances as follows:

- Abscess that occur in the face. The danger triangle of the face is an area encompassing the corners of the mouth to the bridge of the nose. Although rare, it is possible that infections in this area can spread to the cavernous sinus in the brain through the facial veins and cause thrombosis or meningitis.
- In diabetic patients, they may find it difficult to clear the infection.
- If a patient is systemically unwell because of the abscess.
- In immunocompromised patients.
- In the presence of cellulitis.

Cellulitis

This is defined as acute inflammation of the dermis and subcutaneous tissue. Classically it affects those with comorbidities such as obesity, diabetes, and immobility. It affects the elderly with skin that is prone to break after minimal trauma and reluctant to heal.

The common infecting organisms are staphylococcus aureus and streptococcus pyogenes (Group A Streptococcus, or GAS).

The presentation of abscess and cellulitis has been recognised for millennia. The signs were outlined by Celsus in his work *De Medicina* in the first century CE.

- Calor—warm
- Rubor—redness or erythema
- Dolor—pain
- Tumour—swelling (blisters)
- Functio-laesa—loss of function (added by Galen)

Eron classification of cellulitis

Class 1 – No systemic toxicity or co morbidity – can be managed with antibiotic treatment without need for admission

Class 2 – Systemically well or unwell but has **co morbidity** such as obesity, venous insufficiency or peripheral vascular disease or diabetes. These patients will need intravenous antibiotics as short stay for 48 hours followed by outpatient ambulatory antibiotic therapy where available

Class 3 - As above but with a **positive qSOFA** such as tachycardia, hypotension or altered mentation.

Class 4 – Severe life-threatening infection such as **necrotising fasciitis** (based on NICE guidance)

Necrotising fasciitis (NF) is a life-threatening bacterial infection caused by Group A streptococcus and amplified by anaerobic bacteria. The amplification of the original infection occurs because of synergy between the infecting organisms. Therefore, this is also referred to as synergistic gangrene. One of the postulated mechanisms is that the aerobic organisms proceed to cause an anaerobic environment as they invade and inflame the tissues. This secondarily permits the growth of a cohort of anaerobic organisms.

The mortality rate varies from 20 to 40 per cent. From a simple trauma, it can progress very rapidly within hours and lead to sepsis, multi-organ failure, and death.

Necrotising Fasciitis

Type 1: Poly microbial. One set of aerobic bacteria utilise the locally available oxygen and facilitates the growth of a second anaerobic organism causing local thrombosis and haemolysis

Type 2: Group A Streptococcus GAS infection

Type 3: Clostridial infections – causing gas gangrene
If this is suspected a rapid Gram's staining of tissue will help with the diagnosis.

Largely these are clinical diagnoses, but Ultrasound, CT and MRI can help assist the diagnosis if gas locules are noted in the subcutaneous tissue.

Rapid and ruthless excision of all necrotic tissue is the most important part of the management along with critical care management and antibiotic care in consultation with microbiologists

Fournier's Gangrene: Is necrotising fasciitis affecting the perineum and genitalia; whilst it is common in men it can also affect the genitalia in women

Meleney's Synergistic gangrene: affects the abdominal wall after surgery and can be rapidly fatal if not recognised and treated immediately

WOUND HEALING

Surgical wounds heal by first intention when the edges are approximated in the absence of tissue loss in an aseptic environment.

They heal by second intention when there is loss of tissue preventing primary approximation.

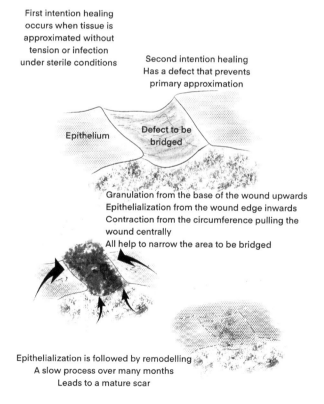

First intention healing occurs when tissue is approximated without tension or infection under sterile conditions

Second intention healing Has a defect that prevents primary approximation

Epithelium

Defect to be bridged

Granulation from the base of the wound upwards
Epithelialization from the wound edge inwards
Contraction from the circumference pulling the wound centrally
All help to narrow the area to be bridged

Epithelialization is followed by remodelling
A slow process over many months
Leads to a mature scar

Figure 36: Wound healing, primary and secondary intention

Where there is tissue loss that prevents primary approximation, the loss of tissue needs to be bridged before the wound heals. These wounds heal by second intention.

This process needs three factors.

- Granulation from the base upwards
- Epithelialisation from the edge that grows towards the centre of the wound
- Contraction, a force that like the spokes of a wheel draws the wound edges towards the centre. Progressively it decreases the area to be bridged by the epithelium.

The process is driven by leucocytes, macrophages, and fibroblasts assisted by angiogenesis

First intention is the healing that occurs after abdominal wounds are closed by approximating the skin. The epithelium being approximated does not need a granulation tissue bridge.

Secondary intention is the healing that occurs when there is loss of tissue and primary approximation of skin is not possible. The granulation tissue then fills the gap, and the epithelium bridges over it.

Phases of Wound Healing

1. **Haemostasis**: This is the process of capillary constriction and platelet plugging to stop bleeding. Meticulous surgical haemostasis contributes significantly to healing.
2. **Inflammation**: Once clots are cleared, the wound is infiltrated by leucocytes and macrophages. Angiogenic stimulation starts.
3. **Proliferation**: Fibroblasts proliferate and encourage glycoprotein and collagen formation. Epithelial proliferation from wound edge is initiated.
4. **Maturation**: Collagen is remodelled, and the wound begins to resemble the surrounding tissue. This process can take up to two years.

Surgical Wounds Classification, NICE Guidance

Clean: An incision in which no inflammation is encountered in a surgical procedure, without a break in sterile technique, and during which the respiratory, alimentary, or genitourinary tracts are not entered.

Clean-contaminated: An incision through which the respiratory, alimentary, or genitourinary tract is entered under controlled conditions but with no contamination encountered.

Contaminated: An incision undertaken during an operation in which there is a major break in sterile technique or gross spillage from the gastrointestinal tract, or an incision in which acute, non-purulent inflammation is encountered. Open traumatic wounds that are more than twelve to twenty-four hours old also fall into this category.

Dirty or infected: An incision undertaken during an operation in which the viscera are perforated or when acute inflammation with pus is encountered (e.g., emergency surgery for faecal peritonitis); for traumatic wounds, if treatment is delayed, there is faecal contamination, or devitalised tissue is present.

Management

Immediate closure can be carried out for clean wounds. They heal by first intention.

Delayed primary closure can be done after a period of 48 hours when treating, clean contaminated wounds and clean wounds that are more than six hours old. After an immediate surgical toilet, these can be left open with a light dressing and then closed forty-eight hours later.

Contaminated and infected wounds are not closed but left open to heal by secondary intention. In these wounds a meticulous wound toilet with excision of all dead tissue and foreign bodies will promote healing by second intention.

This is based on best practice guidelines in disaster situations (WHO 2009).

The introduction of vacuum-based wound dressing has been of great assistance in promoting wound healing and non-messy dressings.

Surgical site infections lead to delay in healing. Winnet Orr, an orthopaedic surgeon, is supposed to have famously said all wounds heal their way to rosy health when left untouched under a plaster cast. Things have moved on since then, and it behoves us to ensure that clean and clean contaminated wounds do not get infected. Infections delay the process of healing and may lead to a longer stay in hospital, and in some situations, they may even delay further treatment like chemotherapy.

Factors That Affect Healing: ABCDEF, and I

A: Anaemia/age
B: Bronchitis—Poor oxygenation, possibly only marginal
C: Cachexia—Poor healing
D: Diabetes—High possibility of infection
E: Emaciated—Poor collagen formation
F: Frailty/fat—Two sides of the same coin
I: Infection—Always to be avoided where possible

POST-OPERATIVE CARE

The length of stay is a key surrogate marker of good care. The stay is lengthened if there are post-operative complications. Complications increase the overall stress levels amongst the carers and the cared. It is therefore necessary to monitor and prevent complications by regular assessment of the patient clinically using physiological parameters. Early detection of abnormal parameters followed by immediate action, is beneficial and puts the patient on the road to a complication-free recovery. It prevents progression down a slippery slope towards increasing levels of care and death in a few.

The daily ward rounds, possibly twice daily for some ill patients, needs to consider all the parameters of the national early warning scores. This must be documented in notes that are timed, dated, named, and signed. The haematological, biochemistry, and radiological results must be noted, and appropriate action taken if needed. The daily fluid balance must be checked. The total intake, output from drains if there are any, and urine output will give an idea of the quantity of fluids that need to be replaced. Timely action on abnormal electrolytes and fluids in the elderly will prevent avoidable cardiac problems such as atrial fibrillation. A review of all medications must be made, with the changes documented. The antibiotic and DVT prophylaxis policy of the hospital must be adhered to.

Pain scores in the NEWS chart must be addressed. The effects of pain on recovery and lung function cannot be overemphasised. Abdominal pain after surgery leads to shallow breathing. The dead space air (residual air from the alveoli to the oral cavity following expiration) has a higher proportion of expired air that is rich in CO_2. Shallow breathing moves the dead space air in and out, leading to a drop in oxygen saturation. Shallow breathing will also fail to fill the alveoli, which may then collapse, leading to atelectasis and/or pneumonia. Intra-abdominal factors for the cause of pain, such as peritonitis or even anastomotic leak, will lead to shallow breathing and a drop in oxygen saturation; it may also be a manifestation of excess opiate analgesia that supresses respiration.

The other effect of pain is tachycardia, and it can have a significant impact on cardiac function, especially in the elderly. With tachycardia, the diastolic period is shortened. Coronary perfusion occurs during diastole, and thus a rapidly beating heart is less well perfused. The implication of this, especially in the elderly and the unfit, is obvious. Tachycardia tires the heart!

Nutrition is an important factor in the post-operative period. With minimally invasive surgery, most patients can start feeding enterally quite early. If it is anticipated that a patient is unlikely to be suitable for enteral feeding for five days or more, then discussions must be had with the nutrition team to decide whether TPN is appropriate. This may well be needed in patients with a bowel fistula or those recovering from peritonitis. In these situations, the ileus is prolonged, and par enteral nutrition may be needed. Albumin, a negative acute phase reactant, is a good indicator of progress. Low levels of albumin do cause oedema of the small bowel, leading to prolonged ileus. It is seldom corrected rapidly by parenteral or enteral protein. Ileus leads to vomiting and some respiratory complications such as aspiration pneumonia. This will certainly lengthen post-operative stay.

The buzzwords are target and trigger.

If hypoxia is noted (more common in the obese, smokers, the elderly, and those with COPD), this must raise the possibility of respiratory problems such as atelectasis in the early post-operative period or infections later. Sepsis and shock of any aetiology and diabetic ketoacidosis must be borne in mind. Hypoxic patients need oxygen. Monitor with pulse oximeter and determine how much oxygen must be given and how.

Blood gases will be necessary if the saturation remains low despite remedial action. If the hypoxia is persistent, the cause of the hypoxia must be determined. At the outset, oxygen is delivered to the maximum possible level in the ward, disregarding COPD. More people come to harm from hypoxia than from the cessation of the hypoxic drive that may manifest as respiratory acidosis and increasing CO_2 levels. Repeat of bloods, ECG, and (if cardiac problems are suspected) troponin levels must be checked. If the problem is purely respiratory in the post-operative period, a CT thorax or a CTPA to exclude pulmonary embolism may be appropriate. An examination of the abdomen along with the chest will exclude subdiaphragmatic mischief, which can manifest as poor respiratory function. A CT scan in those cases will need to include the abdomen and pelvis as a CT TAP (thorax, abdomen, and pelvis).

Post-operative anaemia when present, may need correction with transfusion. The transfusion trigger of 70 g/L may not apply in post-operative states. The targets vary as patients with coronary syndrome post-operatively need a higher level of haemoglobin than a patient with known chronic anaemia. Oxygen carrying capacity is dependent on the level of haemoglobin and the FiO_2. This will need discussions with other clinicians, including the haematologist and the consultant in charge of the patient. The locally agreed policy should be implemented.

Post-operative Complications

Post-operative complications can arise after any operation. Complications arise due to five factors.

- Patient related
- Presenting problem related
- Technique related
- Technology related
- Treatment related

Patient-related complications can arise due to comorbidities and mental status. In elective cases, actions to mitigate these must be taken prior to listing a patient for surgery and at the time of preoperative assessment. Recognition and anticipation of problems due to comorbidities must be highlighted at the 'WHO time out' before every operation. It is now mandatory with the worldwide introduction of the WHO Checklist.

- Diabetic patients, those with hypertension, and those on anticoagulants can be overlooked leading to stress for both the patient and the practitioner.
- Cardiopulmonary exercise testing (CPET) is a surrogate marker for fitness and is useful for anticipating problems.
- The American system of classification into ASA grades 1–5 is useful but subjective. Likewise, the calculation of morbidity and mortality as well as assessment of frailty all remain subjective.
- Mental problems of patients such as one that swallows countless needles or hairpins repeatedly needing many laparotomies may also lead to post operative complications.
- High or low BMI patients are liable to more complications than those in the normal or the overweight range.
- Drug users who present with ischaemic limbs, make reconstructions very difficult which contribute to post-operative complications.
- Ultimately, the matter of proceeding to surgery in a patient that is unfit must be based on discussions with the patient, their family, the surgical, critical care, and anaesthetic teams.

Presenting problem–related complications are sometimes difficult to prevent—for instance the patient who has a faecal peritonitis due to colonic perforation. The operation may be successful, and there may even be no primary anastomosis. Antibiotic cover may be adequate, yet the patient can succumb to overwhelming sepsis. This also applies to patients presenting with peritonitis that follows appendicular abscess or peptic perforation. Preventing it may not be possible as the time of presentation may be too late for a successful outcome.

Anastomoses may break down if the vascularisation is poor or oxygen delivery is decreased due to COPD or cardiovascular pathology despite technically well-fashioned anastomoses.

Technique-related complications can be reduced by regular practice under guidance and seeking assistance when needed. There are many possible complications that relate to technique. A few are highlighted here.

- Repair of a large incisional hernia of the abdominal wall with inappropriate sutures
- Approximating tissue under tension
- Devascularisation during to mobilisation
- Not using the mesh in the proper plane
- Insufficient mobilisation of the bowel for a tension free anastomosis
- Anastomotic technique such as not everting the vascular anastomosis
- Anastomotic technique such as not inverting the bowel anastomosis
- Rough handling of sutures that may fracture later
- Diathermy damage to bowel
- Inadvertent perforation of bowel during laparoscopic procedures or port insertions
- Not placing drains when needed, delaying detection of complications such as bleeding.
- Early post-operative feeding despite the presence of ongoing ileus, leading to problems such as vomiting and aspiration injury to lungs
- Not controlling bleeding at the time of surgery and hoping that the bleeding will stop
- Not checking and ensuring that the procedure has been completed safely

Technology-related complications should be mitigated by attention to detail, but sometimes they may be unpredictable.

- The incomplete firing of a few staples in a stapled anastomosis
- Fracturing of a diathermy needle tip during laparoscopic surgery
- Failure to ensure that the proper gas supply systems are in place for anaesthesia
- Wrong type of operating table, such as one not suitable for a Lloyd Davies position, that prolongs surgery

- Failure of laparoscopic camera/light systems (rare these days)
- Diathermy burn due to improper placement of diathermy pads
- Diathermy injury due to improper setting of the intensity

Treatment-related problems are complications such as the following:

- Bleeding in patients on aspirin or clopidogrel
- Not bridging anticoagulants when needed, leading to post-operative CVA
- Failing to ensure pre-operative medications are prescribed, such as antihypertensives, potassium, digoxin, etc.
- Excessive opiate analgesia leading to sedation and respiratory complications
- Not changing antibiotics based on available results of cultures and sensitivity
- Not considering kidney function in prescribing aminoglycosides and non steroidals
- Not using the appropriate urinary catheter for long term use

This list is only a partial list; there are many such problems that one needs to be aware of always.

The post-operative complications fall into three groups:

- Wound-related complications
- Intra-abdominal complications
- Extra-abdominal complications

The principles of care are universal:

- Systematic examination of the patient
- Examination of the part in concern
- Resuscitation of the patient
- Rapid appropriate investigations
- Timely action

Wound-related complications include wound infection and dehiscence. The infections can be limited to the wound or deep space such as pelvic collections. Where there is a deep wound infection, dehiscence is a possibility. The management follows the first principles laid out earlier and starts with assessment of the patient as a whole and then the part that is affected. Consultation with microbiologists starts at the time of recognition of the infection. Recognition of infection is facilitated by daily ward rounds and attention to detail, including small changes in observations and minor complaints. Would dehiscence is an emergency especially if the bowel is exposed. Where possible intra peritoneal collections must be excluded preferably by a CT scan prior to surgical intervention.

Intra-abdominal complications after surgery commonly involve presence of blood, bile, or faeces; there can also be ischaemia of the bowel or fistula formation due to small or large bowel injury.

Where there is no drain placed after surgery, recognition of any type of collection can be delayed. Changes in the NEWS with respect to oxygen requirement, tachycardia, temperature, and mentation will need evaluation. If necessary, radiological imaging must be arranged after routine bloods that will include CRP, urea and electrolytes, blood sugar, and full blood count.

With ongoing bleeding, the haemoglobin will drop. If there is a drain, then indication for surgery is dictated by the quantity and rate of loss of blood. In general terms, if there is persistent drainage of blood, it is best to group and crossmatch blood prior to return to theatre.

When there is drainage of bile after gallbladder surgery, immediate imaging and discussions with the gastroenterologist will be necessary. The patient may require an urgent ERCP and stenting if bile duct injury is noted. If there is common bile duct injury, the problem needs escalation to a specialist hepato-biliary team. Cystic duct stump leak can be managed with stenting of the common bile duct.

Bile-stained drainage could be due to bowel injury, and as in patients with faeculent drainage, the patient can become rapidly septic. Timely resuscitation will include not only fluids but also antibiotics after sampling blood for culture. Irrespective of the time of day, the patient will need assessment with respect to immediate management, which will include surgical intervention.

Extra-abdominal complications fall into the following general categories:

- Wind related (Lungs): pyrexia from days 0–5
- Wound related: pyrexia from days 5–10
- Water related (UTI): pyrexia from days 10–15
- Wall related (Vein wall): pyrexia from days 10–20

Early pyrexia is mostly due to respiratory problems. Wind and pump complications are related to lungs and heart. The problem with the lung tends to occur early; when early, it is likely to be related to a mucous plug causing atelectasis. The clinical manifestation may only be a drop in oxygen saturation or rise in temperature. Very often these occur in the first couple of days and are best treated with physiotherapy.

Cardiac problems in the post-operative period are generally due to four factors:

- Hypotension and hypovolaemia
- Hypoxia
- Hypokalaemia
- Hypomagnesemia

These should be corrected. Oftentimes, the pre-operative medications such as digoxin and potassium are missed, or the potassium not supplemented.

Wound infections are common after emergency operations for peritonitis. Normally the wounds will show evidence of infection later than two days. A subtle sign may be a slight elevation in temperature. They manifest in a progressive manner as follows:

- Erythema
- Cellulitis

- Serous discharge
- Purulent discharge

Urinary infections may follow the use of catheter. When no direct cause is evident for a patient's pyrexia, urinary infection or line sepsis must be suspected.

Deep wound abscesses can also manifest at this stage and the adage 'Pus somewhere, pus nowhere, pus under the diaphragm' needs to be modified to 'Pus in the body cavities or pus in the lines' such as central lines.

When fever is unaccounted for, all fluids including blood, pus, sputum and urine must be cultured not only for bacteria but also for fungal infections!

Symptomatic deep vein thrombosis in the post operative period can be reduced with preventive measures but even that may be difficult when the cause is pathological such as on-going pelvic malignancy. Thrombo embolic deterrent (TED) stockings are very beneficial, to the extent that one needs to apply these stockings in just seven patients during the perioperative period for one major benefit! The Numbers Needed to Treat (**NNT**) is therefore seven. This is an excellent benefit for such a non-invasive measure. It works by compressing the superficial leg veins thus directing a greater flow to the deep veins of the leg.

It is now unequivocally recognised that after orthopaedic joint replacements and pelvic cancer surgery, some form of anticoagulation for a period of twenty-eight days in the post-operative period is of benefit in reducing the number of patients presenting with post-operative DVT and possibly pulmonary embolism. Patients must therefore be prescribed fractionated heparin or oral anticoagulants (which may prove to be even more beneficial), for this period.

Antithrombotic Medications

Unfractionated Heparin

Heparin acts on the coagulation cascade by inhibiting thrombin (Factor II) and factor Xa. One of the side effects of heparin is HIT, or heparin-induced thrombosis. It thus appears to promote the process that it is supposed to prevent! This is an autoimmune response manifested by decrease in platelet count, thrombosis, and skin allergy. If this is clinically suspected or confirmed, stop heparin immediately, switch to another anticoagulant such as warfarin, and ensure platelet count returns to normal.

Fractionated Heparin—Low Molecular Weight Heparin (LMWH)

This is a synthetic derivative of heparin. Its actions are more predictive and controlled. They are more effective than vitamin K antagonists. Drugs such as Dalteparin, Enoxaparin, and Tinzaparin are now in common usage. They can be used for long periods up to twenty-eight days after major surgical procedures.

Oral Anticoagulants

These include Warfarin, Apixaban, Dabigatran, Edoxaban, and Rivaroxaban.

Warfarin

Warfarin acts as an anticoagulant by inhibiting vitamin K–dependent clotting factors 2, 7, 9, and 10. It also inhibits proteins S and C. Warfarin is usually prescribed for patients with atrial fibrillation or recurrent deep vein thrombosis. Warfarin level can be monitored by regular INR, also known as prothrombin time.

The other newer drugs are described as novel anticoagulants. Unlike warfarin, which can be reversed with vitamin K, for the newer anticoagulants there is no antidote except for dabigatran. Their usage has increased as there is no need for intensive monitoring with INR, as in the case of warfarin and other coumarins.

Reversal of Anticoagulants

Minor bleeding when overt, as from skin injury, is easy to treat with pressure and without long-term consequence.

Major bleeding may not be overt and can be very dangerous with excessive blood loss; the haemoglobin count can fall rapidly.

For minor bleeding with any of the above drugs, desmopressin can be used if simple measures fail. It modulates the levels of factor VIII and VVF. It also increases platelet adhesion.

Where there is major bleeding, then reversal is needed as shown.

Aspirin/Clopidogrel	Platelet transfusion
Heparin	Protamine sulphate with complete reversal
LMWH	Protamine provides partial reversal PCC may be of benefit
Warfarin	Vit K/PCC if needed
Dabigatran	Idarucizumab, 5 g
NOVACS	4 factor PCC

PCC—4 Factor Prothrombin Complex Concentrate

This is a complex of factor II, VII, IX, and X. It is better than fresh frozen plasma but more expensive. It is very useful in major clinical bleeding, especially when surgical intervention is needed. Octaplex is the one of the commonly used complex.

Bridging Anticoagulation for surgery

Many patients scheduled for surgery will be on anticoagulants such as warfarin. Some may be on novel anticoagulants. When elective surgery is needed for patients on anticoagulants, consideration must be given to the need for bridging with low-molecular-weight heparin. It is best to follow the hospital protocol or to discuss with the anticoagulation team. Bridging is needed if, after risk assessment, the risk of thrombo-embolism is high. It is needed in patients who have had the following:

- Venous thrombo embolism (VTE) within the previous three months
- A VTE whilst taking anticoagulants
- AF and TIA within three months
- AF and previous TIA with risk factors such as cardiac failure, diabetes, or hypertension, and the elderly over seventy-five years of age.
- Mechanical heart valves

Deep Vein Thrombosis

Deep vein thrombosis (DVT) contributes to a significant number of preventable deaths. Strict adherence to the identification of persons in need of prophylaxis and implementation of local prevention policies are beneficial. Preprinted risk assessment forms help decrease the risk of DVT.

The following categories of patients are at risk:

- Above the age of sixty
- Smokers
- The obese
- Those with a past history of DVT
- Young women on contraceptives
- Those with varicose veins
- Those with a recent abdominal cancer or orthopaedic lower limb surgery

TED Stockings

These simple stockings do the trick. These stockings offer compression of the calf at pressures of 20 mmhg or less. This compresses the superficial leg veins, the long and short saphenous veins, and therefore directs the flow to the deep veins, thus increasing the rate of flow in the deep vessels. Slowing of flow is one of the triad of pathological changes that lead to deep vein thrombosis.

Prevention and early detection of deep vein thrombosis reduces the risk of pulmonary embolism, which is thought to be as high as 10 per cent in patients with DVT. PE is responsible for 10 per cent of hospital deaths (R. J. Beyth, A. M. Cohen, and C. S. Landfield, *Arch Intern Med* 155, no. 10 [1995]).

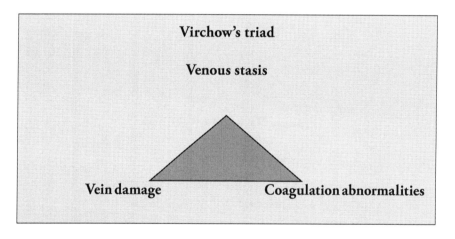

High index of suspicion helps in the diagnosis of DVT, especially in patients with the stated risk factors. Dorsiflexion of the leg, causing pain, is noted in less than 50 per cent of patients (Homan's sign). Phlegmasia cerulia dolens, painful swollen leg, is seldom seen. Commonly there may be redness and swelling. Even so, venograms and duplex Doppler studies are normal in many. If the index of suspicion is high, anticoagulant therapy is advisable at the outset till investigation confirms or confutes the diagnosis.

PE occurs due to clots getting dislodged from the limb veins and moving to the heart and on to the pulmonary artery. This leads to a ventilation perfusion mismatch as areas ventilated may not be perfused due to the absence of blood flow. It imposes a cardiac strain and may manifest initially as reduced oxygenation in post op patients. An ECG may show a normal rhythm in 70 per cent of patients; the classical changes, less commonly seen, are in certain leads referred to as 'S1Q3T3'. More commonly, they present with signs of right heart strain; some have RBBB or even new onset AF. Inverted T waves may be seen across the right heart leads. If the clot is large, then it can lead to death.

If a pulmonary embolism is suspected, it is important to immediately start the patient on high-flow oxygen through a non-breather mask and arrange a CT of the pulmonary artery (CTPA). D-dimer is of little value as it may be raised in the immediate post-operative period. If confirmed, immediate anticoagulation will be needed. Thrombolysis is not likely to be an option in patients who have had major surgery as the risk of bleeding is very high.

Acute Kidney Injury

Acute kidney injury (AKI) is often confronted in the surgical wards.

There are three criteria, three categories, and three stages.

Criteria for AKI

The AKI is an abrupt (within forty-eight hours) reduction of kidney function, manifested by any one of the following criteria.

1. An absolute increase in serum creatinine of 0.3 mg/dL or greater (≥ 26.4 µmol/L)
2. A percentage increase in serum creatinine of 50 per cent or greater (1.5-fold from baseline)
3. A reduction in urine output, defined as less than 0.5 mL/kg/h for more than six hours

Categories of AKI

AKI may be classified into three general categories:

- **Prerenal**—An adaptive response to severe volume depletion and hypotension, with structurally intact nephrons
- **Intrinsic**—Response to cytotoxic, ischemic, or inflammatory insults to the kidney, with structural and functional nephron damage
- **Postrenal**—From obstruction to the passage of urine

While this classification is useful in establishing a differential diagnosis, many pathophysiologic features are shared amongst the different categories.

Staging of AKI

The Acute Kidney Injury Network (AKIN) has proposed a staging system for AKI. In this system, **either** serum creatinine **or** urine output_criteria can be used to determine stage.

Acute Kidney Injury Network Classification/ Staging System for AKI

Stage	Serum Creatinine Criteria	Urine Output Criteria
1	Increase of $\geq$ 0.3 mg/dL ($\geq$ 26.4 μmol/L) or 1.5- to 2-fold increase from baseline	< 0.5 mL/kg/h for > 6 hours
2	> 2- to 3-fold increase from baseline	< 0.5 mL/kg/h for > 12 hours
3*	> 3-fold increase from baseline, or increase of $\geq$ 4.0 mg/dL ($\geq$354 μmol/L) with an acute increase of at least 0.5 mg/dL (44 μmol/L)	< 0.3 mL/kg/h for 24 hours or anuria for 12 hours
*Patients who receive renal replacement therapy (RRT) are considered to have met the criteria for stage 3 irrespective of the stage they are in at the time of RRT.		

Oliguric and Non-oliguric Patients with AKI

Patients who develop AKI can be oliguric or non-oliguric, can have a rapid or slow rise in creatinine levels, and may have qualitative differences in urine solute concentrations and cellular content. Approximately 50–60 per cent of all causes of AKI are non-oliguric.

Classifying AKI as oliguric or non-oliguric based on daily urine excretion has prognostic value.

Oliguria is defined as a daily urine volume of less than 400 mL and has a worse prognosis, except in prerenal injury.

Anuria is defined as a urine output of less than 100 mL/day and, if abrupt in onset, suggests bilateral obstruction or catastrophic injury to both kidneys.

Stratification of renal injury along these lines helps in diagnosis and decision-making and can be an important criterion for patient response to therapy.

Assessment in ARF

- Urine Dipstick for protein/blood
- Urine biochemistry check Na and osmolality
- Urine culture and sensitivity before starting antibiotics
- Renal ultrasound
- CXR to exclude pulmonary oedema
- Non-contrast CT

In pre-renal failure, the kidney is pathologically normal and continues to concentrate the urine. The ability to concentrate the urine means the following on urine examination:

- High osmolality
- High urea
- Low sodium

In intrinsic renal failure or Acute Tubular Necrosis (ATN), obviously the intrinsic renal function is lost and this means the following on urine examination:

- Low osmolality
- Low urea and creatinine
- High sodium
- Presence of casts is typical of ATN

A renal ultrasound may show a normal sized kidney or a small kidney that is less than 9 cm with bright echo in parenchyma. A small sized kidney suggests chronic damage whereas a normal sized kidney is suggestive of acute renal failure, with bright echo due to oedema.

The principles of management are to ensure a tight fluid balance and enable delivery of oxygen to the tubules. This can be done by ensuring oxygen saturation greater than 95 per cent with levels of haemoglobin greater than 7 g/dL.

A further principle is to exclude any toxins that are being prescribed, such as the following:

- NSAIDS
- Aminoglycosides
- ACE inhibitors
- Beta blockers
- Opioids

Cardiac Problems in Surgical Patients

Common cardiac problems in surgical patients are

- hypotension (the most common) and
- tachycardia.

These generally follow from the Four Hs:

- Hypovolaemia
- Hypoxia
- Hypokalaemia
- Hypomagnesemia

Other problems are as follows:

- Primary pump pathology such as myocardial infarction
- Excessive volume infusion

- Changes in rhythm leading to AF
- Pulmonary embolism

As always, absolute values are unreliable than trend over time.

The warning signs that should alert one to the possibility of cardiac complications are as follows:

1. Increased respiratory rate an early marker of the ill patient
2. Progressively decreasing urine output an early marker of poor cardiac output

Urine output is a surrogate marker for cardiac output because a hypoxic kidney cannot work at its best! The medullary nephrons are even in normal conditions working at the boundaries of hypoxia. Any further decrease in oxygen delivery rapidly tilts the balance.

Atrial fibrillation is common in the elderly. Very often, correcting the fluids and electrolytes will enable reversal to a sinus rhythm. It is also likely that the patient's drugs, such as digoxin, (a rare prescription these days) or a beta blocker may have been missed out in the perioperative period and restarting them will assist in rate control.

Tachycardia may be due to hypovolaemia. This will need assessment of the drains for blood loss and adequacy of fluid replacement.

Bradycardia is rare in the surgical patient, and when it occurs, it could be due to pain, beta blocker therapy, or myocardial infarction.

Risk of cardiac problems in non-cardiac surgery patients is proportional to the pre-existing cardiac disease.

High Risk
Recent MI within six months has the highest risk
Unstable angina
Severe aortic stenosis
Decompensated cardiac failure

Uncontrolled hypertension

Cardiac arrhythmia

Lower Risk

MI more than six months ago

Stable angina

Compensated cardiac failure or valve disease

Cardiomegaly

Pacemaker

- All patients with pacemakers need a recent cardiological assessment to ensure pacemaker function prior to surgery
- Diathermy earthing at the time of surgery must be placed away from the pacemaker
- Short bursts of diathermy rather than continuous bouts are preferred
- Bipolar diathermy is safer in these patients than monopolar diathermy

Shock

The definition of shock is an acute circulatory failure leading to inadequate tissue perfusion and cellular hypoxia, cellular damage, dysfunction, and failure of organs.

In the shocked state, autoregulation sets in and directs blood to the kidney and cerebrum at the cost of skin and bowel.

Types of Shock

- Hypovolaemic
- Cardiogenic
- Obstructive
- Vasodilatory

Stages of Shock

    I.   Less than 500 mL blood loss
   II.   500–1,000 mL loss
  III.   1,000–2,000 mL loss
  IV.   Greater than 2,000 mL loss

Hypovolaemia is the commonest cause of shock in surgical patients.

Hypothermia must be avoided because it contributes to bleeding diathesis, as noted in the discussion on the fatal triad.

Exsanguinating patients need immediate definitive action and surgery. Successful resuscitation with 10–20 mL/kg of fluids crystalloids or colloid immediately will improve the outcome.

The type of fluid infused is not as important as the rapidity of action. Crystalloid in excess may cause oedema, whilst colloids can have anaphylactic or allergic reactions. A combination of colloids with crystalloids may be acceptable.

Blood should be given when needed, however if a patient is exsanguinating, it is imperative to control the bleeding before infusing blood, as with ruptured aortic aneurysms or major trauma.

Distribution of fluids between compartments is determined by osmotic forces generated by solutes in the solution. The extracellular fluid is maintained by its cation, sodium (Na). Intracellular fluid is maintained by its cation, potassium (K).

The Na/K/ATPase pump functions to exclude sodium from the intracellular compartment. Water can diffuse across a selectively permeable membrane along a gradient, flowing from an area of higher to a lower concentration along the slope by osmosis. This process helps maintain isotonicity with between the compartments.

The daily fluid intake normally equates to output
Intake: food, water, small amount from metabolism
Output: insensible loss from skin and breathing, sweating, urine and faeces

Daily volume replacement postoperatively must include daily maintenance fluids plus fluids lost from drains and urine

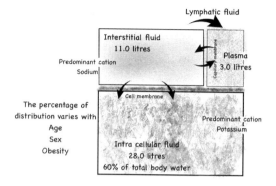

Lymphatic fluid

Interstitial fluid
11.0 litres

Predominant cation
Sodium

Plasma
3.0 litres

Cell membrane

The percentage of distribution varies with
Age
Sex
Obesity

Predominant cation
Potassium

Intra cellular fluid
28.0 litres
60% of total body water

Total body water in a 70 kg adult is 42.0 litres
Total blood volume is 5.0 litres with plasma constituting 60% the rest is cellular

The types of fluid are crystalloids and colloids
Crystalloids diffuse between plasma and interstitial fluid.
They stay where sodium stays

Colloids and blood stay in the plasma
They help to build up volume rapidly

Dextrose and water diffuse through the entire body water
Most useful in replenishing intra cellular compartment in conditions like diarrhoea

Figure 37: Fluid balance

Post-operative Fluid Management

Any major operation will activate the endocrine orchestra led by the pituitary. Prime amongst the various responses, with respect to fluid management, is that major body cavity surgery initiates the ADH-aldosterone system. The antidiuretic hormone does exactly what the name implies: it retains water and sodium.

A reduced urine output immediately after a major operation is a natural response to injury.

Here are some points of note in fluid balance post-operatively.

- Insensible loss is often not appreciated. It can be as much as a litre depending on the presence of fever or the provision of dehumidified oxygen.
- Strict intake output chart must be maintained, and the loss must be replenished over and above the daily requirements.
- Minimally invasive procedures and fast-track recovery will need careful management, as oral fluid regimes may be established early.
- The body retains water and sodium post-operatively.
- Basal water requirement is 30–40 mL/kg/day.
- Daily sodium requirement is no more than 60–100 mmol/day.
- Daily potassium requirement is 40–60 mmol/day. This must not be ignored and must be included from the immediate aftermath of a laparotomy. Overlooking hypokalaemia can lead to cardiac problems.

Enhanced Recovery After Surgery (ERAS)

Recovery is a process that takes time. Individuals recover at different rates depending upon their state of fitness. It is dependent on several factors that include the following:

- Pre-operative health of the patient
- Intra-operative procedural process
- Perioperative care
- Post-operative convalescence

If the problems outlined are assessed and addressed at each point, it is felt that the process of recovery can be accelerated. This has been termed 'enhanced recovery'. Currently, many hospitals have protocols for the patient journey that facilitates recovery.

The pre-operative phase concentrates on the maintenance of optimal health prior to surgery. This includes optimising physical and nutritional fitness by regular exercise and activity, increasing protein intake, and (for colorectal patients) ensuring an adequate carbohydrate load prior to an operation to decrease post-operative insulin resistance. Carbohydrate loading moves the patient to a 'fed' or anabolic state, whereas the previous system of starvation prior to surgery moved patients to a catabolic state. With insulin being an anabolic hormone, the anabolic state sets in prior to surgery with pre operative carbohydrate loading. According to some studies, this preserves insulin sensitivity post-operatively and hastens recovery. This still remains to be proven. Suspending or decreasing smoking and alcohol consumption prior to surgery is beneficial.

Intraoperatively, principles include the following:

- Decreasing bleeding during surgery and using minimally invasive techniques
- Titrating the intravenous fluids to requirement and not 'drowning' the patient with fluids
- Decreasing use of opiates and providing good analgesia by way of epidural or rectus sheath catheters

Post-operatively, the provision of adequate analgesia with epidural or rectus sheath infusion of local anaesthesia facilitates early mobilisation. It allows for sitting at least six hours on day one to standing by the bed and walking with assistance early. This is facilitated by use of fewer tethers such as drains, urinary catheters, and intravenous fluids. Anecdotally in our hospital, walking the patient as soon as possible was contributory to a more rapid recovery. The concept of vertical nursing, whereby a patient is nursed in a sitting position instead of being nursed flat along with daily chest physiotherapy, benefits the lung function. It is worth stressing that the patient must be examined daily by clinicians with assistance from physiotherapists and the pain team. Early introduction of diet must be very carefully titrated by senior clinicians lest it pushes some patients into paralytic ileus.

After discharge, there must be regular communication and coordination with the nursing team. Nutrition, physical activity, and DVT prophylaxis remain key factors.

The rapid recovery process involves less starvation and stress, attention to overall fluid balance, and defined discharge criteria. The policy, when successful, decreases the length of stay.

Cardiopulmonary Exercise Testing (CPET/CPEX)

Cardiac and pulmonary status play a major role in recovery from non-cardiac body cavity surgery. Oxygen demand increases after surgery. An efficient 'pump and pulmonary' system is necessary to deliver this increased demand. The reason for a person's breathlessness may vary from being unfit to having lung, cardiac, haematological, and circulatory problems. Traditional assessment is unable to quantify the cardiopulmonary status as well as the CPET can.

CPET is a non-invasive test that measures the cardiopulmonary status of patients at rest and during exercise.

The actual test commonly involves subjecting the patient to physical exercise on a bicycle or treadmill. The patient breathes through a mouthpiece. This permits concurrent monitoring of oxygen utilisation as well as the carbon dioxide output. ECG, heart rate, and blood pressure are recorded simultaneously. An ECG tracing is done throughout the procedure much like the cardiac exercise testing, and the procedure is discontinued if abnormality is detected on the ECG. The threshold at which the metabolism switches from aerobic to anaerobic metabolism can be calculated; this is the anaerobic threshold (AT).

Anaerobic Threshold

The anaerobic threshold is that point during exercise when the rise in lactate due to exercise can no longer be buffered by bicarbonate. This leads to an increased production of CO_2. At this point, the base excess goes down, and the lactate and CO_2 increase sharply. Technological progress has made it possible to immediately measure this change in gas exchange. Computerisation provides an easy-to-read report.

The oxygen demand goes up after surgery and remains high in the early post-operative period. Knowing the level of activity at which a patient switches from aerobic to anaerobic metabolism will assist in post-operative planning, delivery, delayed delivery, or non-delivery of surgical treatment.

Aerobic capacity is a marker of the ability of the patient to meet the higher oxygen demand that will be necessary after surgery.

Metabolic Equivalents – METS	
Functional Capacity is graded in METS	
Sedentary work	1 MET
Activities of life – climbing/walking	4 METS
Athletic fitness	10 METS
After surgery one is likely to need	>4 METS

The patients who might benefit from this assessment are as follows:

- Patients who are scheduled for major non-cardiac operative procedure
- Patients in need of assessment of lung and cardiac function
- Evaluating recovery for rehabilitation after surgery

The cardiopulmonary exercise test is done a week to two weeks preoperatively, giving time to decide on the type of intervention that will be of benefit to the patient. It must be appreciated that prehabilitation may help improve the performance of some patients and deny surgical treatment to some. Poor functional status can manifest as cardiac problems and increased mortality in the post-operative period. If the patient does not meet the demands that will be needed for a good outcome, discussions regarding risks and benefits of surgery and possible alternative management must be had with the patient.

Older, P. Anaerobic threshold, is it a magic number to determine fitness for surgery?. *Perioper Med* **2,** 2 (2013). https://doi.org/10.1186/2047-0525-2-2

The use of cardiopulmonary exercise testing (CPET) to evaluate cardiac and respiratory function was pioneered as part of preoperative assessment in the mid 1990s. Surgical procedures have changed since then. The patient population may have aged; however, the physiology has remained the same. The use of an accurate physiological evaluation remains as germane today as it was then. Certainly no 'magic' is involved. The author recognizes that not everyone accepts the classical theories of the anaerobic threshold (AT) and that there is some discussion around lactate and exercise. The article looks at aerobic capacity as an important predictor of perioperative mortality and also looks at some aspects of CPET relative to surgical risk evaluation.

This is an excellent review article for those who wish to know more.

Suture Materials and Surgical Technique

The suture materials used for surgery fall into the following categories:

- Absorbable
    - Braided
    - Non-braided
    - Organic
    - Synthetic
- Non-absorbable
    - Non-synthetic
    - Synthetic

The current generation of absorbable sutures are strong and thus have contributed a lot towards replacement of non-absorbable sutures with reduction in 'stitch sinuses' that used to be a complication of non-absorbable sutures such as thread and silk.

Absorbable Sutures

These sutures 'dissolve' over time due to proteolytic action. They do not need removal when used for approximating skin. The story began with catgut made from the mucosa of young sheep (kid) intestine. They are still in use in different parts of the world. The plain catgut gets absorbed in seven days. To make it resistant to dissolution by the proteolytic enzymes of the body, they were chromium coated and labelled 'chromic catgut'. The latter are normally absorbed in twenty-one days. Sometimes they take longer.

Currently in most parts of the world, the absorbable sutures used are synthetic. They are as follows:

- Polyglycolic acid—Dexon
- Polyglactin—Vicryl
- Poly dioxanone—PDS
- Poliglecaprone—Monocryl

These can be used for abdominal wound closures and for approximation of subcutaneous tissue and skin. They may be physically detectable in wounds for up to six months however they lose their strength over time.

The wounds are only half as strong as normal tissue at forty-two days after surgery, and they are 90 per cent as strong as the normal for that patient in six months. They are also weakest at eight days, the time when traditionally patients used to be discharged. In patients with recurrent laparotomies, it may be preferable to offer them external support such as an abdominal corset for up to six weeks after surgery.

Non-absorbable Sutures

Non-absorbable sutures are used when it is important to ensure that the wounds remain stronger for longer. One needs to reflect on the fact that approximating paper with steel will only tear the paper! In the final analysis, it is the nature of the tissue and the process of healing and degree of mechanical support that will determine the strength of the wound. The sutures merely bring edges together so nature can build a bridge.

Commonly used non-absorbable sutures are as follows:

- Polypropylene
- Polyester
- Nylon
- Silk (rarely used now)

Surgical Technique—Handling of Tissue

Gentle handling of tissue with graceful movement along embryological planes during laparotomy and minimal loss of blood promotes recovery. It is often quoted that the surgeon must have the eye of an eagle, the heart of a lion, and the hand of a lady. Delicacy in handling tissue cannot be overemphasised.

Some useful basic principles from my routine teaching of surgical technique are presented here:

Handle with tact, not force	Brutal force only tears tissues, rendering dissection more difficult.
Always protect the needle tip	This principle must always be adhered to.
Needle tip at 90 degrees to the surface that is being engaged	Positioning the needle tip at 90 degrees will provide maximum mechanical advantage. With a curved needle that is engaged at 90 degrees, the tip will egress at the other side on just a gentle forward pressure.
Protect and poke	When approximating the abdominal wound, it is important to protect the underlying bowel loops from injury during the inward stroke. This is done by using the back of the forceps against the under surface of the sheath through which the needle is inserted.
Pick and poke	During the outward stroke, the sheath is pulled upwards and away from the contents. The needle tip is engaged against the sheath at 90 degrees on the under surface.
Follow the yellow brick road	The principle here is, 'Find the plane, and the job's a game.'
Embryological planes	These are non-vascular, such as the lateral peritoneal fold mobilisation during colectomy. Find it, and then you can move gracefully, bloodlessly, and harmlessly along this plane.
Pathological planes	This can be vascular or strong when fibrosed and needs careful dissection.
Traction, countertraction, and action	This will help in defining the embryological plane and also assists in dissection of the pathological plane. Without traction (always gentle but constant) and sustained progress, the plane will be lost.

Traction close to action	Traction faraway from the site of dissection is pretty well useless.
Too much traction is distraction	This is true as if tissues are pulled apart instead of dissected, and then the plane is lost with bleeding.
Blood fogs the plane	If there is minimal bleeding, the plane is seen throughout the procedure and will greatly facilitate dissection.
Follow the foam	During dissection, with gentle traction, areolar tissue will be seen; this is very obvious during laparoscopic surgery but also clear during open operations. By following the 'foam', the chance of 'straying away from the field' is less.
Never lose sight of a hot tip	As a 'hot tip is a dangerous tip'. This applies particularly to laparoscopic procedures, when the diathermy tip remains hot after use and should not be moved away from the field of vision of the camera. It must be watched all the time.
No tension no break down	As in life, so in surgery. Where there is tension, there is breakdown. Holding things together with forces that wish to move away never helps.
Do not have blood on your hands	The lesser the blood loss, better the recovery.

MULTIPLE CHOICE QUESTIONS—TEST YOURSELF

1. A sixty-five-year-old man is unable to do routine work but can take care of his activities of daily living. His WHO performance status is:
   a. Two
   b. Zero
   c. One
   d. Three
   e. None of the above

2. You are called to assess an elderly lady with cellulitis in the leg. After assessment, you conclude that the patient could be in a state of sepsis because:
   a. She has a temperature of 37.9 degrees with a painful inflammation in her right foot.
   b. Her respiratory rate is 22/minute, and her systolic blood pressure is 85 mmHg.
   c. The pain in the leg is very severe, and she needs more analgesics.
   d. She is walking about with a limp because of the inflammation.
   e. She says it started with a thorn prick when she was gardening.

3. Patients with septic shock can be identified by:
   a. A systolic pressure of 95 mmHg or less.
   b. Persistent cough for more than two days.

c. The need for intravenous fluids to maintain a MAP of 100 mmHg and a lactate of 3 mmol/L.

d. Need for vasopressors to maintain a MAP of 65 mmhg or greater and a lactate of 2 mmol/L or less.

e. Need for vasopressors to maintain a MAP of 70 mmhg or greater.

4. A fourteen-year-old boy presents with pain that started in the umbilicus the previous evening. At the time of the ward round, he has severe pain in the right lower quadrant of the abdomen. Appendicitis is diagnosed. The reason for the change in location of pain is:

   a. Increased flatulence at the time of onset.

   b. Inflammation of the appendix at the tip and not the base of the appendix.

   c. Inflammation of the parietal peritoneum extending to the visceral peritoneum.

   d. Inflammation of the visceral peritoneum extending to the parietal peritoneum.

   e. Somatic pain proceeding to autonomic pain.

5. An eighty-two-year-old lady presents with acute onset of pain and tenderness in the right iliac fossa, suggesting appendicitis. Actions prior to consideration of surgical intervention must include:

   a. Assessment for fitness for surgery

   b. CT scan to exclude carcinoma of the caecum or other pathology

   c. Discussion with the anaesthetist

   d. All of the above

   e. None of the above

6. At laparotomy for a right iliac fossa mass thought to be due to appendicitis, the surgeon finds a thickened distal ileum with a normal caecum. The options include:

   a. Suspect Crohn's disease and proceed to biopsy a lymph node

   b. Appendicectomy

   c. Suspect tuberculosis and proceed to an appendicectomy

d. Suspect that it is a Meckel's mass and proceed to resection of small intestine

e. Suspect Crohn's disease, biopsy a lymph node for diagnosis, and do an appendicectomy

7. What are the possible positions where the appendix can be located?
   a. Pelvic
   b. Retro-colic
   c. Paracolic
   d. Pre- or post-ileal
   e. All of the above

8. At operation for appendicectomy, a Meckel's diverticulum is noted in the distal small bowel. The complications of Meckel's diverticulum include:
   a. Bleeding
   b. Perforation
   c. Obstruction
   d. Peritonitis
   e. All of the above

9. An eighty-four-year-old patient is admitted with features of acute appendicitis. Six hours later, the patient's temperature is 38.5°C, heart rate is 106/min, and respiratory rate is 24/min. The white cell count is 15.0 x 10^9/L and CRP is 160. On examination, she is tender all over the abdomen. The cause for the rapid progression is because:
   a. She is elderly
   b. She is constipated.
   c. The omentum is attenuated and localisation has failed.
   d. Previous hysterectomy has prevented localisation.
   e. She has cystitis.

10. A sixty-five-year-old man presents with a history of nausea and upper abdominal discomfort for a few weeks. On examination, he has clinical jaundice with a non-tender palpable mass in the right upper quadrant of the abdomen that moves with respiration. Based on the clinical finding, you suspect:
    a. Acute cholecystitis
    b. Acute pancreatitis with subhepatic abscess
    c. Common bile duct stones causing jaundice
    d. Pancreatic malignancy
    e. Hepatic flexure carcinoma

11. A sixty-three-year-old man presents with jaundice and upper abdominal pain. An ultrasound confirmed the presence of multiple small gall stones, but the common duct could not be visualised. MRCP showed a CBD that was 12 mm dilated with a possible impacted stone at the ampulla. The management is:
    a. Proceed to a MRCP
    b. If MRCP shows a common duct stone, perform a ERCP and extraction of calculus
    c. Check coagulation status prior to ERCP
    d. Warn the patient about possible complications of ERCP, including pancreatitis
    e. All of the above

12. The Murphy's sign is important when assessing acute cholecystitis. It is dependent on the location of the fundus of the gallbladder which is:
    a. At the tip of the right ninth costal cartilage in the trans pyloric plane
    b. At the tip of the left ninth costal cartilage along the mid axillary line
    c. Parallel to the umbilicus on the right
    d. In the right flank
    e. Immediately to the right of the xiphisternum

13. Following a difficult laparoscopic cholecystectomy on a seventy-four-year-old man with previous history of pancreatitis, there is evidence of bile-stained discharge of over 350 mL on the second post-operative day. Your options are:
    a. Examine the patient clinically, exclude peritonitis, and request urgent bloods and liver function tests.
    b. Arrange immediate imaging CT or US.
    c. Discuss with gastroenterologist and arrange an urgent ERCP and stenting, if needed.
    d. Inform the patient that you suspect injury to the bile or cystic duct.
    e. All of the above.

14. A week after a day case laparoscopic cholecystectomy, a fifty-four-year-old lady presents to the acute surgical unit with jaundice. Clinically, the abdomen is soft. She has no tenderness. The full blood count and CRP are normal. Bilirubin is 90, and alkaline phosphate is 160. Rest of the liver function tests are normal. The most likely diagnosis is:
    a. Injury to the common bile duct
    b. Injury to the cystic duct
    c. Injury to the liver
    d. Movement of small stones to the CBD during laparoscopic dissection
    e. Hepatitis

15. A thirty-nine-year-old lady presents with typical features of biliary colic. The ultrasound examination has failed to demonstrate any abnormality in the gallbladder or liver. The liver function tests and routine bloods are normal. A CT scan of the abdomen is also normal. She continues to have transient post prandial pain lasting for up to six hours at times; it is always located in the right upper quadrant. There is no change in bowel habit and no bloating to suggest irritable bowel. The next step could be:
    a. Reassure and discharge the patient.
    b. Ask her to see if she can come to terms with the discomfort.
    c. Prescribe buscopan as an antispasmodic.

d. Arrange a HIDA scan of the gall bladder.

e. Ask her to take Proton pump inhibitors daily.

16. A sixty-year-old lady has pelvic pain. The gynaecologist arranged an ultrasound scan of the abdomen. It shows normal adnexal and pelvic contents but has picked up multiple stones in the gallbladder. She is referred for surgical opinion regarding the next step.

    a. Discuss operative and non-operative options with the patient regarding management of asymptomatic gallstones.

    b. Advice immediate laparoscopic cholecystectomy.

    c. Manage expectantly and repeat ultrasound scan in six months.

    d. Arrange a CT scan.

    e. Reassure and discharge her.

17. A previously fit sixty-three-year-old man presents acutely with clinically detected jaundice. He has no abdominal symptoms. The full blood count shows the following: Hb, 144g/L; WBC, 11.9 x 10⁹/L; bilirubin 160, alkaline phosphatase, 240. AST is normal. On examination, the abdomen is non-tender, and there is no palpable abnormality. Ultrasound examination has shown tiny gallstones, but the CBD could not be visualised due to overlying bowel. The jaundice could be due to:

    a. Stones in the CBD impacted at the lower end

    b. Stones in the cystic duct

    c. Hepatitis

    d. Pancreatitis

    e. Hepatic flexure carcinoma

18. A fifty-eight-year-old man presents with a three-day history of increasing pain in the left lower quadrant of the abdomen. He does not have pyrexia. There are no urinary symptoms. He has been passing flatus. On examination he, is very tender in the left the lower abdomen. Routine bloods show a WBC count of 20.0 x 10⁹/L. Provisional diagnosis is acute diverticulitis. The next step is:

    a. A CT scan of the abdomen

    b. Urgent laparotomy

c. MRI of the pelvis

d. Laparoscopic examination of the abdomen

e. Supine abdominal X-ray

19. A seventy-seven-year-old man presenting with abdominal pain and tenderness has a CT scan that shows a large localised pelvic collection without evidence of free gas. There is evidence of diverticulosis in the left colon. The radiologist reports that this is a localised diverticular abscess. The options for further management could be:

a. Drainage under imaging control

b. Proximal colostomy and drainage

c. Laparoscopic lavage and drainage

d. Hartmann's procedure

e. Any of the above

20. A seventy-three-year-old lady who had a low anterior resection eight days ago is increasingly unwell. The oxygen saturation is 94 per cent and the heart rate is 110. The NEWS score is 7. The CXR on day seven was normal. On examination, her abdomen is distended and tender. She has had one loose bowel movement. The clinical diagnosis that must be considered is:

a. Pneumonia

b. Post-operative cardiac event

c. Atelectasis

d. Anastomotic leak

e. Bowel obstruction

21. A sixty-five-year-old man had a coronary artery bypass graft four days ago. The operation was difficult. He has been started on fibre-rich enteral feeding on day two. He now has a distended abdomen that is non-tender. He is not passing flatus. A supine abdominal X-ray shows dilated colon and small bowel. His haematological and biochemical parameters do not suggest sepsis. You arrange a CT scan, and that rules out mechanical obstruction. The radiologist reports it as a possible pseudo-obstruction. The management is:

a. Intravenous fluids

b. Correction of electrolyte imbalances

c. Endoscopic decompression and exclusion of mechanical cause

d. Surgical decompression if refractory, to conservative management

e. All of the above

22. A seventy-five-year-old man had repair of bilateral inguinal herniae laparoscopically. He returns with abdominal pain, tenderness, and vomiting forty-eight hours after surgery. Supine abdominal X-ray shows distended loops of small bowel with pockets of extraluminal gas. The possible diagnosis is:

a. Inadvertent bowel injury

b. Retained carbon di oxide causing distension

c. Analgesics causing constipation

d. Recurrent hernia

e. Eating very soon after surgery

23. Five days after a total colectomy for ulcerative colitis in a thirty-nine-year-old lady, her progression is slow. This is attributed to the steroids that she had been on prior to surgery for acute colitis. The abdomen is tender. The stoma is dusky. WBC was 16 x10^9/L two days previously and now it is 25.0 x10^9/L. Platelet count is 35.0 x10^9/L. CRP is 215. The possible cause of this deterioration is:

a. Increasing opiates for pain

b. Previous steroid therapy

c. Not continuing the antibiotics

d. Paralytic ileus

e. Ischaemic stoma and distal small bowel

24. A fifty-three-year-old lady presents with adhesive obstruction following a hysterectomy when she was thirty-nine years old. At operation, she needed resection of the terminal ileum and a right hemi colectomy with release of other adhesions in the proximal bowel. Five days later, she remains distended and has not opened her bowels or passed flatus. Her abdomen is not tender, and she has not needed opiates for the last two days. Hb is 123. WBC is 13.5. Albumin is 18. She is apyrexial. What is the probable cause?

a. Paralytic ileus
b. Bowel injury
c. Anastomotic leak
d. Pelvic abscess
e. Intra-abdominal bleeding

25. A forty-two-year-old male with a strong family history of carcinoma colon is referred on the fast track with looseness of stools and a positive FIT test. The quantitative analysis is 210 mcg/g. The next step in management is:
a. Reassurance that he is too young to have a serious problem.
b. Arrange an ultrasound scan of the abdomen
c. Arrange an immediate colonoscopy and prescribe bowel prep.
d. Arrange a CT scan.
e. Arrange a flexible sigmoidoscopy within three months.

26. A forty-two-year-old lady presents with aches and pains in both wrists, right knee, left hip, and lower back. She complains of increasing tiredness and thirst. She has lost 10.5 kg in one year. The serum calcium has been elevated on three repeated tests; albumin is normal. Ultrasound scan shows a 21 mm × 15 mm complex solid nodule just deep to the right lower lobe of the thyroid gland. Rest of the neck is normal. The possible diagnosis is:
a. Parathyroid hyperplasia
b. Parathyroid adenoma
c. Thyroid nodule
d. Vascular haemangioma
e. Prominent pyramidal lobe

27. A forty-nine-year-old lady with ultrasound-detected parathyroid adenoma confirmed on a Sestamibi scan is likely to have:
a. A low corrected serum calcium
b. A high corrected serum calcium
c. A low parathormone level
d. A high calcitonin
e. An elevated serum phosphate

28. An eighty-year-old diabetic lady has severe abdominal pain six days after an anterior resection. On assessment, she has a temperature of 38.4°C, a pulse rate of 98/min, a respiratory rate of 24/min, and a poor urinary output. Oxygen saturation is 87 per cent on 100 per cent oxygen delivered through a non-rebreathing mask. What is the most likely cause for her tachypnoea?
    a. Opiate analgesia prescribed for pain
    b. Increased delivery of oxygen
    c. Intra-abdominal sepsis leading to metabolic acidosis
    d. Poor control of blood sugar post-operatively
    e. Massive intra-abdominal haemorrhage

29. A thirty-two-year-old alcoholic presents to the surgical assessment unit with a six-hour history of vomiting and abdominal pain. On assessment the pulse rate is 98/min; respiratory rate 22/min; oximetry shows 92% saturation. The abdomen is very tender with guarding in the epigastrium. Chest X-Ray is normal. The WBC count is 16.3 10^9/L. Serum amylase is 956 and CRP is 88. The possible diagnosis is:
    a. Gastritis
    b. Right basal pneumonia
    c. Cholecystitis
    d. Hepatitis
    e. Acute pancreatitis

30. One day after a major laparotomy for intestinal obstruction you are requested by the surgical high care to write up a fluid regime. The base line requirement over 24 hours for a 70 kg man is likely to be:
    a. Three litres of normal saline with 20 mmol of kcl/litre
    b. Two litres of normal saline with 20 mmol of kcl/litre and one litre of 5% dextrose saline
    c. Three litres of dextrose saline with 20 mmol of kcl/litre
    d. One litre of normal saline and two litres of 5% dextrose with 20 mmol of kcl in each litre
    e. One litre of gelofusin and two litres of 5% dextrose with 20 mmol of kcl/litre

31. A fifty-seven-year-old male presents with severe abdominal pain and vomiting of twelve hours duration. A clinical diagnosis of acute pancreatitis is made. The severity of the disease can be assessed by which of the parameters?
   a. Glasgow score of 14 or more
   b. C reactive protein > 150
   c. Elevated serum amylase
   d. Elevated serum bilirubin
   e. Body mass index > 30

32. Which of the parameters in the above patient would indicate the need for ERCP and sphincterotomy?
   a. Serum bilirubin of 130
   b. Serum amylase of 1120
   c. CRP of 300
   d. WBC count of $16.0 \times 10^9/L$
   e. Serum calcium of less than 1.4

33. A twenty-nine-year-old man presents with abdominal pain of eight hours' duration. There is no history of previous pain, and he is not on any medication. On clinical examination, the abdomen is rigid, and he is in a state of systemic inflammatory response syndrome. The patient continues to deteriorate and is scheduled for surgery as he is found to have free gas in the erect chest X-ray. The anaesthetist requests a blood gas analysis. It is likely to show:
   a. PaO_2 of 20 mmHg
   b. Respiratory acidosis
   c. High bicarbonate
   d. Elevated base excess
   e. metabolic acidosis

34. An eight-four-year-old lady presents to the emergency ward with upper abdominal pain of twenty-four hours and pyrexia. On examination, she is tender in the upper abdomen. A diagnosis of acute cholangitis is made as she is jaundiced. Biochemical investigations are likely to show
   a. Mostly elevated unconjugated bilirubin
   b. High Conjugated bilirubin

c. Normal bilirubin

d. Low CRP

e. Normal alkaline phosphatase

35. A seventy-two-year-old man presents with dry gangrene of his right big toe. Diabetes has been eliminated as the cause. Previously, he had an angioplasty of the right superficial femoral artery with some improvement in his symptoms. The foot is warm. Dry gangrene is characterised by which of the following factors?

    a. A clear line of demarcation between the gangrenous and non-gangrenous tissue

    b. Presence of cellulitis proximal to the gangrenous toe

    c. Presence of infection in the toe

    d. Watery discharge

    e. Purulent discharge

36. The gangrenous toe in the above patient needs to be treated by which of the following options?

    a. An immediate bypass graft

    b. Urgent medial compartment fasciotomy

    c. Lateral fasciotomy

    d. Symptomatic relief and elective amputation, if necessary

    e. Fore foot amputation is preferable because it heals well

37. A thirty-year-old woman presents with severe diarrhoea and vomiting of one day's duration. The water loss that follows is:

    a. Likely to be from both intra- and extracellular compartments

    b. Likely to be in the extracellular compartment

    c. Generated by osmoreceptor activity in the pituitary

    d. A parasympathetic activity is responsible for repletion of water

    e. Likely to be greater in the intracellular compartment

38. A forty-five-year-old lady with a body mass index of 32 presents with a history of intermittent upper abdominal pain mainly located in the right upper quadrant of the abdomen. The pain was first noticed at the outset six months ago after dinner and kept her awake for most of

the night. It settled by the morning but has recurred intermittently. She has had no fever. On examination the abdomen is soft and non tender. She is likely to have:

a. Acute cholecystitis
b. Acute cholangitis
c. Biliary colic
d. Crohn's disease
e. Renal colic

39. A forty-year-old man has a lump in the back overlying the scapular region on the right for over ten years. The lump has been slowly increasing in size. It is not painful. It is 10 cm in length, 7 cm in width, mobile, and non-tender. The skin over it is healthy, and there is no evidence of any punctum.
The most likely diagnosis is:

a. Subcutaneous lipoma
b. Epidermoid cyst
c. Pilonidal cyst
d. Hidradenitis
e. Carbuncle in the back

40. A sixteen-year-old lad presents with pain in the left shoulder and left upper quadrant of the abdomen following an injury to the abdomen while playing football. He was seen in the A&E and sent home with paracetamol. He returns the following day with more pain. The Hb is 100 g/dL, and the HR is 114 and blood pressure 100/60mmhg. A splenic injury is suspected. A CT scan is likely to show:

a. A capsular tear with a subcapsular haematoma
b. A complete laceration of the spleen with massive intra abdominal haemorrhage
c. A ruptured kidney
d. A lacerated bladder
e. A Perforated colon

41. Post-splenectomy protocol consists of:
    a. Immunisation against encapsulated bacteria
    b. Antibiotic prophylaxis for life
    c. Recognition that severe infections are most likely to occur in the first two years after splenectomy
    d. Implantation of splenic tissue into the omentum after traumatic splenectomy
    e. All the above

42. A seventy-seven-year-old man presents to A&E in a state of collapse. A FAST scan shows the presence of free fluid and an aortic aneurysm. He is resuscitated with fluids and the systolic blood pressure is maintained at 100mmhg. The CT scan confirms the presence of a ruptured abdominal aortic aneurysm (AAA) of 6.6 cm indicating the need for an immediate open repair. His quality of life is good, and his performance score is 1. In the past, he has had a myocardial infarction with placement of a stent. At operation, as the infrarenal aorta is cross clamped, his blood pressure drops to a systolic of 70mmhg. This is due to:
    a. A sudden increase in after load
    b. An Increase in preload
    c. Acute renal failure due to blood loss
    d. Hypoxia
    e. Not having taken his usual medications

43. In the above patient, on completion of the operation, the aortic clamp is released, and this establishes flow to the distal segment. On declamping the aorta on the operating table, there is the possibility of:
    a. Hypotension
    b. Hypertension
    c. No change in blood pressure
    d. Hypoxia
    e. Renal failure

44. A fifty-seven-year-old diabetic patient presents with a progressive painful left foot. On examination, the big toe is dusky, and there is an area of cellulitis around it. He has no sensation around the distal foot. The popliteal pulse is palpable, and the lower leg feels warm. His HbA1C is 58. What is the possible diagnosis?
    a. Wet gangrene
    b. Dry gangrene
    c. Femoral embolism
    d. Diabetic nephropathy
    e. Popliteal aneurysm

45. A nine-year-old boy presents with acutely worsening pain in the lower abdomen on the right. He had been to school in the morning, but the parents were called at lunchtime because he was vomiting and complaining of pain. On examination, the abdomen is normal with no areas of tenderness. The pain is increasing, and the WBC count is 15 10^9/L. The next step is:
    a. Examine the scrotum and rule out a testicular torsion
    b. Check the urine for infection
    c. Examine the spine
    d. Examine the hips
    e. Reassure his parents and discharge him

46. A thirty-three-year-old man is seen in the acute surgical unit with a painful lump in his natal cleft. He is hirsute and has a BMI of 35. On examination, he has a red and tender swelling in the upper part of the natal cleft. The likely diagnosis is:
    a. Ischiorectal abscess
    b. Fistula in ano
    c. Pilonidal abscess
    d. Perineal haematoma
    e. Abrasion and inflammation

47. A twenty-seven-year-old man presents with an acutely painful left testis of twelve-hour duration. He has had dysuria for two days. The management involves:
    a. Urgent Doppler scan of the scrotum to exclude torsion of testis
    b. Urine dip stick to check for nitrites
    c. Urine dip stick to check for sugar
    d. Consideration of a diagnosis of Epididymo orchitis
    e. All of the above

48. A thirty-nine-year-old lady presents with severe colicky pain in the right loin for twelve hours. It seems to be radiating to the groin. The urine dip stick is negative for nitrites but positive for blood. What is the possible diagnosis?
    a. Ureteric colic due to an oxalate stone
    b. Ureteric colic due to a triple phosphate stone
    c. Renal failure
    d. Cystitis
    e. Dysmenorrhoea

49. A previously well forty-nine-year-old man presents with a painful swelling in the perineum that has been progressive over two days. There is no change in bowel habit and no history of rectal bleeding. On examination, there is induration with tenderness in the ischiorectal fossa area on the left. This is likely to be:
    a. A Perianal abscess
    b. Anal Crohn's
    c. Pilonidal sinus
    d. Perianal haematoma
    e. Acute haemorrhoids

50. MRSA infections are due to:
    a. Streptococcus pneumoniae
    b. Staphylococcus infections that are sensitive to penicillin
    c. Streptococcus infections resistant to methicillin
    d. Staphylococcus infections resistant to methicillin
    e. Multi-resistant streptococcus

51. A sixty-year-old lady presents with acute abdominal pain and vomiting of eight hours' duration. The serum amylase and lipase are raised. She is known to have gallstones. The abdomen is tender. Pancreatitis is diagnosed. Corrected serum calcium is 1.2. Which of the following is correct?
    a. Low calcium is due to poor intake of milk
    b. High calcium is a good prognostic sign
    c. Amylase digests fat and is elevated, suggesting fat necrosis and low calcium
    d. Lipase digests fat, and low calcium is a marker of fat necrosis
    e. Low calcium is not an indicator of severity

52. A fifty-eight-year-old man has pancreatitis. The severity of the presentation can be graded by the Glasgow criteria if:
    a. Three or more factors are abnormal at forty-eight hours
    b. Two or more factors are abnormal
    c. If a patient over fifty-five presents for the first time with pancreatitis
    d. If the amylase is more than three times normal limit
    e. If the PaO_2 is 96 per cent

53. Eight weeks after being treated for pancreatitis, a patient presents with being unwell. There is no pyrexia or vomiting. On examination, he has a large non tender mass in the upper abdomen.
    a. This is likely to be a pseudo cyst of the pancreas.
    b. This is a pancreatic abscess.
    c. This is likely to be a gastric outlet obstruction.
    d. This is typical of a mucocoele of the gallbladder.
    e. This could be acute gastric dilatation, and the patient needs an urgent nasogastric tube insertion.

54. A pseudo-pancreatic cyst:
    a. Is a cyst around the pancreas that is walled off by adjacent structures.
    b. Is a pancreatic cyst that is lined by epithelium of the columnar type.
    c. Is an organised haematoma.

d. Is a distended duodenal diverticulum.

e. Never resolves spontaneously.

55. A sixty-three-year-old lady presents with nonspecific upper abdominal pain. Clinical parameters are normal, and the abdomen is not tender. Seven years ago, she had cholelithiasis, for which she had an ERCP and sphincterotomy followed by a laparoscopic cholecystitis. Gastroscopy was normal, and CT scan shows air in the biliary tree and a dilated common bile duct. What is the cause of air in the biliary tree?

a. Clostridial infection

b. Anaerobic gas–forming organism, causing infection

c. Previous sphincterotomy

d. Laparoscopic cholecystectomy in the past

e. Biliary fistula

56. A seventy-three-year-old lady presents with bilateral pedal oedema acutely. Duplex scan of the legs did not show DVT. Non contrast CT scan of the abdomen shows bilateral hydronephrosis and a retroperitoneal mass. The serum creatinine is 312, and urea is 22. She immediately needs what?

a. An urgent laparotomy

b. Bilateral stenting of the ureters

c. Catheterisation of the bladder

d. Laparoscopy

e. CT Urogram

57. A seventy-four-year-old man with a history of CVA three months ago presents with bowel obstruction. He has had no abdominal operations in the past. CT scan of the abdomen shows a small bowel obstruction caused by a band. Options for management include:

a. Discussion with anaesthetist regarding suitability for surgical intervention

b. Considering the discontinuation of anticoagulation if any

c. Weighing the risk of intervention with further complications of CVA

d. Gastrograffin orally to evaluate need for surgical intervention

e. All of the above

58. A CT scan in an eighty-three-year-old man presenting with obstruction confirms left colonic obstruction with a distended caecum greater than 15 cm. The patient's performance score is zero. He is not on any medications other than pantoprazole. The management is:

a. Wait and watch progress over forty-eight hours

b. Colonoscopy and confirmation of diagnosis

c. Urgent laparotomy

d. Liquid paraffin orally

e. Stenting the area of stenosis

59. A sixty-nine year old lady on warfarin for AF presents with acute obstruction confirmed on CT scan. Ischaemic bowel is suspected. The INR is 3.6. What should be considered prior to surgical intervention?

a. Discussion with haematologist regarding reversal prior to intervention surgically

b. Vitamin K orally for three days with regular monitoring of INR

c. Stop warfarin for forty-eight hours prior to intervention

d. Stop warfarin and bridge with clexane for forty-eight hours

e. Cryoprecipitate infusion prior to surgery

60. An eighty-year-old lady with dementia presents with lower abdominal pain, distension of abdomen, and a palpable mass in the left groin. Supine X-ray of the abdomen shows distended small bowel loops. What should be done?

a. A best interest meeting to determine further management

b. An urgent laparotomy to relieve obstruction

c. Analgesics and antibiotics intravenously

d. Non-operative management

e. PEG to assist with nutrition

MULTIPLE CHOICE
ANSWERS

1. **A.** If a person is able to take care of their daily activities but finds working difficult the score is 2. It is worthy of note that the patient is active for more than 50 per cent of the day. Increasing scores denote decreasing performance. As the performance decreases, the physiological response to injury of any type decreases. Frailty as a person ages is a good determinant of suitability or otherwise for major interventions.

2. **B.** qSOFA is a quick method of assessing the possibility of organ dysfunction and sepsis and enables early recognition. The qSOFA is a bedside method for rapid identification in the ward or primary care setting of adult patients with a focus of infection that when positive indicates poor outcome. qSOFA is positive if two of the three parameters that follow are identified: a respiratory rate of 22/min or greater, altered mentation, or systolic blood pressure of 100 mm Hg or less.

3. **D.** Mean arterial pressure (MAP) is defined as one-third of the pulse pressure added to the diastolic pressure. The pulse pressure when the BP is 120/80 is the difference between the systolic and diastolic, 40. MAP is therefore 83 (80 plus 13.3). The new definition of septic, simply put, is that once the volume is repleted, if a vasopressor is needed to maintain a MAP of 65 mmHg and a lactate of 2 mmol/L, the patient is deemed to be in septic shock.

4. **D.** As discussed earlier, the migrating pain of appendicitis is driven by the depth of inflammation. At the outset, the inflammation involves the visceral peritoneum that is tightly enveloping the appendix. Progression of inflammation involves the parietal peritoneum. This increase in severity is manifest by move to an area of somatic nerve innervation from an area of autonomic innervation. Visceral to parietal. Autonomic to somatic.

5. **D.** Image before invasive intervention. CT scan is more sensitive and has a greater positive predictive value than an ultrasound scan. Depending on availability and feasibility, use of CT scan reduces negative appendicectomy or removal of the 'lily white' appendix that used to be common when wholly based on tenderness at McBurney's point or the Psoas test. CT scan has the drawback that it exposes younger patients to radiation and insult of contrast. Imaging before invasive intervention has now become acceptable for acute appendicitis as it avoids needless intervention and defines alternative pathology such as malignancy and tubo-ovarian disease. B. Reich, T. Zalut, and S. G. Weiner, 'An International Evaluation of Ultrasound vs. Computed Tomography in the Diagnosis of Appendicitis', *Int J Emerg Med* 4, no. 8 (2011)

6. **E.** Imaging before invasive surgery will avoid this scenario, however imaging is not universally available. Controversy exists in these situations, if appendicectomy should be done when Crohn's or TB is noted. TB normally involves the caecum, but Crohn's has skip lesions that may be noted at surgery. If the caecal base is macroscopically normal, it may be safe to proceed to an appendicectomy. The histology must be checked post-operatively. There may be a small risk of a fistula in any operation for Crohn's disease. Current trends do not favour immediate resection as medical management may obviate the need for surgical resection in Crohn's where preservation of bowel is of paramount importance.

7. **E.** Retro-colic and pelvic positions are the commonest. Pre- and post-ileal are the least common.

8. **E.** Meckel's diverticulum, it is often stated, is present in 2 per cent of the population, is two feet from the ileocaecal valve, and has two complications. Bleeding and obstruction. Bleeding when it occurs is due to ulceration at the tip of the diverticulum, and often in these situations, there is a separate blood vessel from the mesentery reaching across the bowel from the mesenteric border. If any young person has melaena and the gastroscopy and colonoscopy are normal, one must exclude Meckel's. I have done with gratifying results on three occasions!

9. **C.** In the very young, the omentum is undeveloped, and in the very old, it is atrophied. The omentum is a phenomenal organ that is referred to as the 'abdominal policeman'. It seeks areas of mischief and contains it by wrapping around areas of inflammation. If it is underdeveloped, the process of containment fails leading to the spread of inflammation. The absence of containment must also be borne in mind in patients who are immunocompromised and those on steroids.

10. **D.** This classically supports the Courvoisier's law. In these patients, the gallbladder is clearly palpable, much like a mucocoele would, the only difference being that this patient is jaundiced. A double impaction of a stone in the cystic duct and another in the CDB may also cause findings similar to this, as would a Mirrizi.

11. **E.** It is important in jaundiced patients to check the coagulation profile prior to ERCP. In some, the malabsorption of vitamin K can affect the coagulation.

12. **A.** This surface marking is quite important when examining a patient suspected of having acute cholecystitis. In general terms, surface marking relates to bony structures than soft tissue as adiposity and aging are confounders.

13. **E.** When there is bile in the drain, sepsis must be suspected. This patient has a drain, but in situations where there is no drain and the patient presents unwell a couple of days after laparoscopic cholecystectomy, it is expedient to proceed to a CT scan followed by drainage and

ERCP. The key principle is that patients must progressively improve daily after laparoscopic surgery. When the recovery is not progressing as per expectations, immediate intervention with imaging and even laparoscopy is indicated.

14. **D.** During laparoscopic cholecystectomy, there are times when small stones are noted in the cystic duct as it is being dissected or clipped. In those cases, when the stones in the cystic duct are appreciated, it is best to milk the stones back to the gallbladder and clip the cystic duct distal to the stones.

15. **D.** Hepatobiliary iminodiacetic acid (HIDA) scan. This involves injecting a radioactive tracer intravenously. This is taken up by the liver cells and excreted into the bile ducts and intestine. The bile with the radioactive tracer collects in the gallbladder if the cystic duct is patent. On detecting a full gallbladder, the patient is given a fatty meal (a Mars bar or sandwich). The gallbladder, in response to a fatty meal, must contract and empty the contents to the intestine. If there is delayed emptying or lack of emptying, it may suggest a physiological dysfunction. The problem may relate in some to a hold up by gravel in the spiral valves of Heister, that represents mucosal folds in the cystic duct. A few patients reproduce their symptoms.

16. **A.** This situation is not uncommon. When the gallstones are asymptomatic, the decision to proceed to a laparoscopic cholecystectomy versus expectant management is often an informed decision by the patient. An argument can be made for a laparoscopic cholecystectomy in a fit young patient because of possible complications over time. This may not be the case in an unfit or elderly unfit patient. The final decision to proceed to a cholecystectomy must be a joint decision with the patient after clear documentation of the discussion.

17. **A.** Common things are commoner and rare things are rarer. One must try to fit the findings to one diagnosis when it is staring you in the face. Multiple diagnoses are more common as one ages! Here, the presence of tiny stones in the gallbladder obviously favours the suggestion that

some of these stones may have moved to the cystic duct. Pancreatic cancers may present with similar biochemical abnormalities.

18. **A.** CT scan is very useful in determining the extent of the disease. Is it just an inflammation, or is it a pericolic, or a paracolic collection, or generalised peritonitis with free fluid? Each one of these can be manged differently. If peritonitic, the distinction between faeculant and purulent may be difficult purely on imaging, and in fit patients, immediate surgery is needed.

19. **E.** The type of treatment offered to every patient is dependent of the individual circumstances. All these options need consideration. In certain situations, a laparoscopic drainage with a more definitive elective resection at a later stage may obviate the need for a stoma which a Hartmann's will certainly require. In some, a stoma may be altogether the best option for the patient.

20. **D.** Whilst all the other options are feasible, anastomotic leaks tend to occur between day four and day eight. Respiratory and cardiac problems occur earlier. A drop in oxygen saturation at any stage must be taken seriously and investigated thoroughly. It is also the harbinger of poor cardiac function and often leads to poor renal function, as the nephrons deep in the medulla do not take kindly to decrease in oxygen levels because they are normally functioning at the limits of oxygen delivery.

21. **E.** This situation is not uncommon. Often the cause is unclear, but it is essential to exclude electrolyte abnormalities. I have seen this after early introduction of high fibre diet in some patients but this is anecdotal. Endoscopic decompression is of great value and may need repetition. It helps to exclude unrecognised mechanical factors such as coincidental stenosis or malignancy.

22. **A.** Bowel injury after transperitoneal laparoscopic hernia repair, though rare, tends to occur. The key principle here is that if a patient fails to progress after laparoscopic operation of any type, especially after day case operations, one must ensure adequate assessment and

investigation. These may include further laparoscopy or imaging prior to intervention. The key message here is not to ignore the patient who returns with symptoms following day case laparoscopic surgery.

23. **E.** A raised white cell count, low platelet, and elevated CRP in a post-operative patient, especially one that is on steroids, must raise the suspicion of ongoing sepsis and the need for imaging and assessment prior to intervention. A dusky ileostomy may be evidence of full thickness ischaemia and die back ischaemia of the terminal ileal segment within the abdominal cavity. This will require re operation and formation of another stoma with good blood supply.

24. **A.** Paralytic ileus is likely when the pre-operative period has been protracted and optimal nutrition has not been possible. Whenever a patient is assessed as ebing unlikely to start feeding within five days of surgical intervention, it is best to discuss nutritional supplementation parenterally at the outset.

25. **C.** Age is not a consideration to delay investigations in the presence of evidence of red flag signs. A FIT test, when positive, must be investigated thoroughly prior to exclusion of pathology leading to it.

26. **B.** A single nodule in the presence of this history is suggestive of an adenoma rather than hyperplasia. Adenocarcinoma is also possible but it is very rare (1 per cent of cases). When it is a single adenoma, successful minimally invasive surgery will provide rapid relief of symptoms. Further biochemical monitoring till return to normal is mandatory.

27. **B.** Parathormone drives the calcium out of the bone by increasing osteoclastic activity. It is a disease categorised by 'bones, stones, groans, and psychotic moans'!

28. **C.** Acidosis and sepsis go together. Seldom, if ever, do we see metabolic alkalosis in surgical post-operative patients. Oxygen debt is the prime cause of metabolic problems. When there is tachypnoea, there is

shallow breathing and recirculation of dead space air that is richer in CO_2 than O_2.

29. **E.** In acute pancreatitis, the amylase rises rapidly within six hours; it also falls rapidly thereafter and is not a measure of severity. In some patients with severe alcoholism, there may be prior pancreatic insufficiency, and the amylase may not be elevated. In patients with peritonitis, ischaemic bowel, and ectopic pregnancy, the levels can be raised. Normally when the level rises to three times the normal value for your lab, pancreatitis is most likely.

30. **C.** The sodium retention after surgery usually means that the baseline requirement of sodium is only 90 mmol a day. This is adequately provided by three litres of dextrose saline. Each litre contains 31 mmol of sodium. It is a combination of half normal saline (0.18 per cent Na) and 4 per cent dextrose. A litre of normal saline contains 154 mmol of sodium; Ringer Lactate and Hartmann's solution contains about 130 mmol of sodium. The baseline potassium is 60 mmol per day, and this is often forgotten, leading to low potassium and cardiac arrythmias in some elderly patients.

31. **B.** CRP is a good indicator of prognosis. The point to note here is that serum amylase, however high the level, is not an indicator of severity.

32. **A.** Patients with acute pancreatitis should have an ERCP with sphincterotomy within seventy-two hours if they have jaundice, cholangitis, or a dilated CBD. Sphincterotomy with stent placement is needed in the presence of cholangitis to allow for drainage.

33. **E.** Metabolic acidosis is a manifestation of oxygen debt and sepsis. In the presence of cellular hypoxia, there is a shift from aerobic to anaerobic respiration leading to the production of lactic acid and a marked decrease in ATP. The acid (H^+) enters the red cells, which contains the enzyme carbonic anhydrase. The bicarbonate buffer reacts with hydrogen very rapidly in the presence of the catalyst, carbonic anhydrase, and forms carbonic acid (H_2CO_3). The carbonic anhydrase catalyses H_2CO_3 in a reaction that can proceed reversibly

in either direction to $HCO_3 + H^+$ or to $H_2O + CO_2$. The excess acid is converted to carbonic acid and then to H_2O and CO_2. Respiratory rate increases to blow off the excess carbon dioxide.

34. **B.** Conjugated and water-soluble bilirubin. It is conjugated with glucuronic acid, a fatty acid to form a salt.

35. **A.** Dry gangrene has the following characteristics: there is a line of demarcation, the demarcation line is aseptic, and the gangrenous area is shrunk and shrivelled.

36. **D.** Generally, immediate intervention is not likely to be needed in this patient as the foot remains well perfused. Assessment for critical limb ischaemia must be made along with a referral to vascular team.

37. **A.** When the body loses water, in situations like cholera, fluid is usually depleted from both the extracellular and intracellular compartments. A range of compensatory responses come into play, leading to stimulation of the renin-angiotensin-aldosterone system and activation of the sympathetic system to preserve the body fluid volume and retain the sodium. Changes in osmotic pressure lead to stimulation of osmoreceptors in the hypothalamus that increases thirst. In conditions like haemorrhage, the extracellular fluid (ECF) volume is decreased selectively. This in turn causes a fluid shift from the intracellular compartment (ICF) to the ECF. The body-to-brain messaging attempts to preserve the interior milieu with many tricks. The immediate activation of the sympathetic system is the major player, as it struggles to maintain the cardiac output and falling blood pressure. It shifts the fluid within compartments and increases the venous tone and heart rate. Renin angiotensin mechanism comes into play and helps to retain sodium and water. The latter is a slower process than the former.

38. **C.** Biliary colic is a misnomer in that the pain can last for many hours unlike a typical intestinal colic that lasts for just a few minutes. It is highly likely that the pain occurs due to movement of gallstones when the gallbladder contracts in response to a fatty meal. The stones may then get impacted in the cystic duct causing pain. As

the gallbladder relaxes later, the stone falls away from cystic duct with relief of symptoms. These types of patients are best undergoing cholecystectomy at the same admission. It avoids the possibility of recurrence, further admissions and harm during the waiting period.

39. **A.** The presence of a lump with a palpable edge that slips under the palpating hand and mobile in all directions makes it likely to be a lipoma. Lipomata can be at located at various levels such as subcutaneous, subfascial, intramuscular, and submuscular, but a subcutaneous lipoma is mobile in all axis. Neurofibroma in the subcutaneous plane are also mobile but only in one axis, and that is perpendicular to the direction of the nerve from which it arises. Epidermoid or sebaceous cysts, in contrast, are not mobile because they are in the intradermal and not the subcutaneous plane. Any lump that is mobile is therefore unlikely to be an epidermoid cyst.

40. **A.** A small capsular tear with a contained subcapsular haematoma can be difficult to diagnose clinically. The history should alert one to the possibility of a splenic injury. In young people, most splenic injuries can be managed conservatively if the patient remains haemodynamically stable. Repeat radiological assessments can be by ultrasound examination, but the primary investigation needs to be a CT scan with grading of the type or rupture. Even in adults, splenic tears up to grade 3 may be managed non-operatively if haemodynamical stability is maintained.

41. **E.** Patients who undergo splenectomy are at increasing risk of overwhelming sepsis, possibly for life. The risk is greatest in the first two years after splenectomy. The risk of infection from capsulated organisms such as H. influenzae, strep. pneumoniae, and N. meningitidis dictates the need for vaccination against these, preferably at the time of discharge from the hospital. Antibiotic prophylaxis with penicillin/Erythromycin is recommended for life.

42. **A.** These patients are 'arteriopaths', as very seldom does vascular disease affect a single vessel in isolation. Despite being able to carry on activities of daily living, an imposition of additional strain on

the heart is likely to affect the cardiac function. A left ventricular ejection fraction of greater than 30 is beneficial for recovery from this type of surgery that requires cross-clamping of the abdominal aorta. With cross-clamping of the aorta, the heart is suddenly placed under increased strain against which it must pump. This can lead to immediate decompensation.

43. **A.** On declamping of the aorta, there is a sudden outflow of blood to the peripheries. The distal tissue would have been hypoxic during the period of cross-clamping, and on reperfusion there is a release of products of metabolism into circulation causing peripheral vasodilatation. This leads to a fall in blood pressure referred to as declamping hypotension and possible injury to the kidneys leading to acute tubular necrosis. Volume loading the patient prior to declamping and gradual establishment of flow distally, such as declamping one limb at a time, may be of assistance.

44. **A.** Typically in wet gangrene as opposed to dry gangrene, there is no clear zone of demarcation. The transition zone between the area with no blood supply and area with some blood supply in wet gangrene is referred to as a zone of septic separation. The fact that popliteal pulse is present shows that diabetes is a disease of the small vessels. Absence of sensation is due to diabetic neuropathy.

45. **A.** In young boys who present with acute lower abdominal pain, the examination of the abdomen is not complete unless the scrotum is examined. When the abdomen is non-tender in the presence of increasing pain, one must exclude torsion of the testis and renal colic.

46. **C.** Pilonidal sinus is common in the hirsute individuals with a high BMI. During the Korean War, this used to be common amongst young GIs and was referred to as 'the Jeep bottom'. The hair in the sinus is always directed so that the root of the hair is superficial and the tip deep, indicating that the hair is from extraneous sources.

47. **E.** The dictat used to be that acute testicular pain in the young adult is likely to be due to infection and in the child due to torsion. There

are always exceptions to the rule, so it is mandatory to exclude torsion in all acute testicular pain with an immediate Doppler scan.

48. **A.** Oxalate stone is also called a 'mulberry calculus' after its resemblance to a mulberry seed that is tiny and spiculated. As this stone moves down the ureter, it abrades the transitional epithelium of the urinary tract and causes microscopic bleeding. The triple phosphate stag horn calculus, however, is soft and smooth and creeps up on the patient asymptomatically and at times even bilaterally.

49. **A.** Perianal abscess may present without the typical fluctuation that is seen in abscesses. There is normally induration. Acute tenderness in this region dictates examination under anaesthesia that will normally include an incision and drainage along with a rectal examination to document the presence or absence of an internal opening of a fistula in ano. Fistula in ano is commonly associated with perianal abscess. A culture swab must be taken. Staphylococcal infections suggest a cutaneous origin. Presence of E. coli or klebsiella raises the possibility of a fistula as the cause of the abscess.

50. **D.** Methicillin-resistant Staphylococcus aureus (MRSA). These are a type of staphylococcus that is resistant to many of the antibiotics commonly used to treat patients with staph infections. They tend to occur in the community or in healthcare settings. Healthcare workers may contribute to transmission in healthcare settings; infections may follow invasive procedures increasing complications and length of stay. Vascular grafts and joint replacements may be infected by MRSA, leading to increased morbidity and even mortality. In community-acquired infections, the spread is by skin contact.

51. **D.** Lipase is the enzyme that digests fat. With pancreatitis, the exocrine digestive enzymes are released into the peritoneum. These are protease, which digests protein to amino acids; amylase, which digests carbohydrates to disaccharides such as glucose; and lipase, which digests the fat. The end products of fat digestion are fatty acids and glycerol. The fatty acids bond with calcium and form soap. The

substrate for lipase to act upon is the fat around the pancreas and the omentum, and this can manifest as fat necrosis. A decrease in calcium level is therefore a sign that indicates severity of the pancreatitis.

52. **A.** Classically, the severity of pancreatitis is assessed based on laboratory findings. The reason for the assessment of is to ensure that the patient gets the appropriate treatment at the appropriate level of care. When the severity index is positive on laboratory and clinical findings, the mortality rate can be as high as 30 per cent.

53. **A.** A pain-free lump more than six weeks after pancreatitis is likely to be a pseudocyst rather than an abscess. In this patient, there is no vomiting, and that rules out a gastric outlet obstruction. Abscesses present earlier and are tender. A pseudocyst is encysted and walled off by the surrounding tissue. Some cysts may communicate with the pancreatic duct, and these may resolve without intervention. The management of pseudo-cyst is dependent upon the findings on imaging. If the cyst is thick walled and it fails to resolve with conservative management, it can be drained endoscopically. When it is multiloculated and fails to resolve, it may need surgical drainage.

54. **A.** As noted earlier, the pseudo-cyst is walled off by surrounding structures. As such, the lining is mesothelial and not epithelial.

55. **C.** In the presence of a sphincterotomy, air from the intestines can be seen in the biliary tree. The biliary duct is open to the duodenal contents. This can cause cholangitis on occasion. The biliary ducts do not have smooth muscles. Once it is dilated, for whatever reason it always remains dilated.

56. **B.** This lady needs immediate treatment from the point of view of the failing renal function. Subsequent assessment needs to be made regarding the cause of the retroperitoneal abnormality. The distinction is between a lymphoma and retro-peritoneal fibrosis. The latter is better defined whilst a lymphoma is irregular in structure and outline. Contrast imaging is contraindicated because of the poor renal function.

It is not recommended unless it can be followed by immediate renal filtration.

57. **E.** The feasibility of an operation is not an indication for its performance. In most cases, however, we need to make a careful assessment of the benefits versus the risks of surgery and discuss the management with the patient and his surrogates.

58. **C.** In this patient's case, because he is fit, an urgent laparotomy is the best course to adopt. In certain situations where the patient may not be fit for surgery but suitable for intervention, endoscopic stenting can be considered. However, gas needs to be instilled during colonoscopy. This may lead to further distention, perforation, and peritonitis.

59. **A.** This patient will need to be discussed with a haematologist because surgical intervention may be required soon. It is not appropriate to wait for forty-eight hours because the obstruction may worsen. Reversal may require the use of Octaplex.

60. **A.** These are difficult situations, and a decision needs to be taken on an individual basis. It is mandatory to make an assessment of risk versus benefit with regard to surgical intervention. This discussion must be had with surrogates, especially in the presence of lack of capacity on the part of the patient.

REFLECTION ON SENTINEL MOMENTS IN SURGERY

Surgical history, it has been said, can be divided into two phases: before Lister and after Lister. Pasteur proposed the germ theory, but it was Lister who made the link between sepsis and germs. Surgery of today stands on the foundations laid by great intellectuals who observed and made links that changed the world. The list here is an incomplete acknowledgement to the contributions made by many to change the face of surgery, over the last few hundred years. It is a salutation to those who got us to where we are now.

Ambroise Pare (1510–1590), the renowned French surgeon, ran out of hot oil, which used to be the prevailing method of dressing wounds in battle. He had to switch to water and egg yolks. To his astonishment, the wounds healed with less pain and suffering. He realised that dressing wounds with boiling oil was detrimental to wound healing and that using a soothing agent produced better results. Thus, by a combination of serendipity and observation, he changed the concept of wound dressing forever. He did not accept the power of authority when it conflicted with his observation.

William Harvey (1558–1657) was the first to describe systemic circulation based on the preparatory work of others. Until his time, Galen's concept of blue blood being made in the liver and red in the heart was popular. According to this, all the blood that was made was consumed by the body on a daily basis. Imagine how much must have been produced and destroyed daily! Harvey calculated that this must be in hundreds of litres every day! He concluded that blood must be recycled. He spent most of his life in elucidating the concept of blood flow, and he carried out painstaking dissections and established that blood in the veins always flowed towards the heart. Understanding of recycling of blood and proving it in those times was no easy task. He showed that the heart pumped the blood to the rest of the body through the systemic circulation, and the blood then passed through capillaries and returned through the venous system. This made a phenomenal contribution to the progress of knowledge.

Antonie Van Leeuwenhoek (1632–1723), the father of microbiology, was one of the first users of microscope. He designed his own microscopes and used them to examine fluids. He was amazed to find little creatures moving about with flagella. Until then, there was no realisation that there were microscopic creatures. He called these creatures 'animalcules', or little animals. He saw bacteria, spermatozoa, and even red cells and muscle fibres. He wrote about his findings to **Robert Hooke**, who was the president of the Royal Society in London. Hooke did not believe it initially, till he sampled water from the river Thames and noted they too were crawling with animalcules!

Ephraim McDowell (1771–1830), a surgeon in Danville, Kentucky, is credited with carrying out the first body cavity surgery by operating on Jane Todd on Christmas Day 1809. He had been called to visit her by her family doctor who thought she was pregnant. She lived miles away, and the home visit was a day's work that took him on horseback over hours of travel through dangerous Native American territory. He concluded that Jane was not pregnant but had a tumour in the pelvis. He advised her of the findings and suggested that if she were to come to his house in Danville, he would remove it, little expecting her to come. To his surprise, she did, and he removed a 22.5 kg ovarian tumour on a table in his living room! It must have been benign because she outlived the surgeon and died many years later of old age. The operation was done without anaesthesia, without relaxation, and without sterilization in the living room of the surgeon in Danville! The only drawback was that it left her with an incisional hernia.

William Morton (1818–1868) anaesthesia was 'born' on the 16 October 1846. Prior to that, All surgery was limited to rapid smash and grab. Surgery was mostly related to amputations. On this day in 1846, John Bigelow, a surgeon in Boston, Massachusetts, arranged for the removal of a tumour from the neck of Edward Abbott by the sixty-eight-year-old Professor Warren. Morton, a young man, had heard of the use of ether from magicians and dentists. He worked on a system of delivery and arrived late to the theatre even as Warren was about to give up, calling all this a hoax! Morton gave anaesthesia to the young man and then turned to the surgeon and said, 'Your patient is ready!' The anaesthesia with ether worked, and the patient felt no pain during the surgery, which lasted for forty minutes. At that moment, surgery was transformed. Professor Warren realised the impact of this and declared, 'Gentlemen, this is no hoax!' Science, it is said, took control of pain on that day. Simultaneously, in 1847 in Edinburgh, **James Simpson** was working on chloroform anaesthesia. Queen Victoria decided to have chloroform anaesthesia for her second delivery. Once the queen decided to have it, the rest of the public clamoured for it, and it became a status symbol.

Louis Pasteur (1822–1895). Prior to his studies, it was believed that life arose spontaneously. Whilst studying the process of fermentation, he was able to prove by simple experiments that distilled fluid did not spontaneously grow organisms unless contaminated by dust and air. He laid the foundation for germ theory.

Ignas Semmelweis (1818–1865), in Vienna, also noted that hand washing reduced the mortality simply by observing the differences in practice between the first and second clinics in Vienna. In the first clinic, medical students delivered the babies. In the second, midwives delivered the babies, and the mortality from puerperal sepsis was much lower. People used to beg to go to the second clinic for fear of death. It so happened that the medical students had anatomy dissections in the morning, and from there they came to the delivery room in the afternoon. Semmelweis's friend Jakob Kolletschka, a pathologist colleague, accidentally cut his finger during the post-mortem of one of the women who died of puerperal sepsis. He too died of sepsis. Semmelweis attended that post-mortem. It showed the same changes of puerperal sepsis noted in previous post-mortems. Semmelweis did not know of germ theory but recognised that if hands were washed, then puerperal sepsis would be lower. He introduced chlorine hand washing, and puerperal sepsis rates fell. He wrote a paper on this for an European journal. It was turned down and he was condemned for even suggesting that the nurses had cleaner hands than the doctors! Finally, after a study in Dublin reconfirmed his findings, it was proven that handwashing saves lives! The tragedy is that Semmelweis was hounded out of Vienna and went back to Hungary, where he died three days after being confined as a lunatic.

Joseph Lister (1827–1912) made great progress in the control of post-operative wound infections. He was aware of Pasteur's work and had heard about carbolic acid being used to clean sewers. Hand washing was still not popular despite Semmelweis's study. Infections were believed to be due to 'miasma', or bad air, but after Pasteur, it became clear that germs caused infections. He used carbolic acid spray during operations and cleaned instruments with it. There was a drammatic reduction in infections and death. He used to begin his operations by saying, 'Let us spray.' A carbolic acid spraying machine would then be started in the theatre before all his surgeries. His success, like that of the proverbial apple of Newton, is reported to be an event when a young boy with a compound fracture of the leg was treated with carbolic acid dressing. When bones were exposed in wounds in those pre-antibiotic times, it meant certain death. Lister applied layers of gauze soaked in carbolic acid. The boy recovered fully, and the era of antisepsis was born. He was a meticulous researcher. He made the link between germs and infection and led surgery towards antisepsis and asepsis.

Robert Koch (1843–1910) made great strides in transmission of infectious disease, especially tuberculosis, which was very prevalent in his times. He showed that to prove that an organism causes disease, four principles must be established, referred to as the Koch's postulates:

- **Isolate**—the organism from the infected person
- **Infect**—reintroduce the isolate into animal models

- **Reproduce** the symptoms
- **Confirm**—repeat the culture and confirm that it is the same organism

He was thus able to show that tuberculosis was caused by mycobacterium tuberculosis, and he received the Nobel prize for his studies.

Alexander Fleming (1881–1955). Serendipity favours the prepared mind. Fleming was a keen researcher and noted that a fungal contaminant had inhibited the growth of a colony of staphylococcus. His paper in 1929 was acted upon by Chain and Florey in Oxford in 1941. With the help of Heatley, the active ingredient, penicillin, was transferred to water, enabling large-scale production and treatment of infection in 1945. Many soldiers were saved in the last year of World War II because of penicillin. The antibiotic era, a process by which one biological substance inhibits another, was born and changed the management and control of infections forever.

Karl Landsteiner (1868–1943) distinguished the blood groups in 1901 and then, with Wiener in 1937, the Rhesus factor. He found that blood of two people, when combined, agglutinates. He separated the factors and called them A, B, and O. The O group contains no antibodies, and O negative is therefore a universal donor. A small proportion of patients with the AB group can accept blood groups A, B, or O and are thus universal recipients. He found that blood transfusion was possible between people with same groups, opening the way for large-scale blood transfusion.

William Bovie (1882–1958). It was known that electric current over certain frequencies could cut tissue without harming the surrounding area. Bovie used this principle to make the first electro-surgical device to control bleeding during surgery. Working with Harvey Cushing, he used the instrument to remove a vascular brain tumour. The impact of this is immeasurable in modern surgery.

William Halsted (1889–1922) was an American surgeon who made a major contribution to breast cancer surgery. Having trained in Europe, he had learnt the European technique of using carbolic acid. The theatre sister, Caroline Hampton, whom he married, developed contact dermatitis to the carbolic acid. Halsted contacted the Goodyear Rubber Company and asked them to design a glove for use in theatre. This, in addition to all the other progress, ushered in a new era of asepsis. Today, no one would think of operating without washing their hands and wearing gloves!

Aspirin, aka acetyl salicylic acid (1899). Pharmaceutical company Bayer developed aspirin from salicylic acid which was derived from willow bark and known to have pain relieving properties. German chemists working for Bayer, Felix Hoffmann and Arthur Eichengrun added an acetyl group to salicylic acid and the now world-renowned aspirin was born. The name aspirin was coined by Bayer and the A stands for acetyl and 'Spir' because salicin is derived from the plant Spiraea ulmaria. 'in' was a suffix for medicines. Bayer, scientists also developed Heroin another great opiate analgesic.

Minimally invasive surgery. The contributions of many to minimally invasive surgery has currently transformed the face of surgery. Operations that required inpatient stay for days have become day case surgery, leading to massive reduction in the number of hospital beds. With the improvement in technology that is still evolving rapidly, the impact is felt not only on the length of stay but also more importantly in the reduction in the level of patient discomfort. Here, I will acknowledge just a few, but do reflect on the fact that progress has been made in small steps by interventions of the many. Prime amongst the changes that facilitated endoscopy and laparoscopy are the following:

- A rod lens telescope
- Strong light source—the 'cold light', which is pretty hot!
- System to deliver light from a distance—fibreoptic glass cable
- A video camera that is miniaturised
- Television screen

What a transformation this progress has achieved in the latter half of the last century!

Harold Horace Hopkins (1918–1994) was a renowned British physicist who introduced the rod-lens system for laparoscopy. His inventions are in daily use throughout the world. These include zoom lenses, coherent fibreoptics, and the rod-lens endoscopes, which opened the door to modern minimally invasive surgery.

Karl Storz (1911–1996), concurrently with the progress in fibreoptic glass technology in the United States and Japan, developed the fibreoptic 'cold light' source. **George Berci,** a urologist, pioneered minimally invasive urology and brought together **the lens and the light** in the early 1960s. Glass fibre technology was imported, and Storz termed his light source the 'cold light'. Now, a light source could be powerful and placed farther away from the site of surgery. In the early days, I recall using light bulbs at the ends of rigid scopes that would all too often fuse at the wrong time! Views were limited by the available brightness. With this immense improvement, the tubes were all light and all the visible structures bright!

Kurt Semm (1927–2003) was a German gynaecologist and is rightly labelled as the father of laparoscopic surgery. In the 1970s, he was made to undergo a brain scan by his colleagues in Kiel University, Germany, because his colleagues felt only a person with brain impairment could perform such surgery. He introduced laparoscopic oophorectomy and tubal ligation. In 1980, Semm performed the first minimally invasive appendicectomy.

In 1982, the first solid state camera was introduced.

In 1987, Phillipe Mouret performed the first video-laparoscopic cholecystectomy in Lyons, France. The improvement in video camera and light technology and introduction of imaging technology in the 1980s, with the advent of ultrasound, CT, and MRI scans, has changed the face of surgical care and permitted changes in endoscopy, early detection, and less invasive management of many disease.

Treatment of patients, despite all these changes, should be guided by standard principles because any deviation from the norm can lead to disaster.

When King Edward VII was being treated for cor pulmonale by Bertie Dawson of the London Hospital, he asked how he proposed treating him. 'Sire,' replied Dawson, 'I shall treat you like any of my patients in the wards at the London Hospital.'

Sir Robert Hutchison (1871–1960). I conclude with the famous quote from the British physician whose methods in clinical examination were most favoured in the twentieth century prior to the advent of imaging technology. This is universal and applicable today and always.

> From inability to let well alone, from too much zeal for the new and contempt for what is old, from putting knowledge before wisdom, science before art and cleverness before common sense, from treating patients as cases and from making the cure of the disease more grievous than the endurance of the same, good Lord deliver us.

ABOUT THE AUTHOR

He has considerable experience in teaching and training junior doctors and surgeons. He served as the Postgraduate tutor (Hospital Dean) for the Blackpool Teaching Hospital and was a member of the Northwest deanery education committee. He was also the chair for the Lancashire and Cumbria network for colorectal cancer.

He has served the Royal College of Surgeons of England as an examiner and Trainer for over two decades assisting with courses such as the basic skills and Care of the Critically ill surgical patients (CCrISP) where he is also a director. He is an examiner for the MRCS.

INDEX

Printed and bound by CPI Group (UK) Ltd, Croydon, CR0 4YY